Susi's presentation is simple to understand and very clear.... This is a great book and will be helpful for teachers and serious students.... I think Anatomy and Asana should be on required reading lists for yoga teacher training programs. It has tremendous value as an anatomy primer!

— *Margot Kitchen, Senior Iyengar Teacher*

Anatomy and Asana:
Preventing Yoga Injuries

by Susi Hately Aldous

First Edition

Text copyright © 2004, 2006 by Susi Hately Aldous
Illustrations copyright © 2004, 2006 by Paulette Dennis

Published by **Eastland Press**
P.O. Box 99749, Seattle, WA 98139, USA
www.eastlandpress.com

U.S. and international sales:
Eastland Press
1240 Activity Drive, #D
Vista, CA 92081
www.eastlandpress.com

Canadian retail sales:
Functional Synergy Press
102, 6323 Bowness Road NW, Calgary, Alberta T3B OE4
www.anatomyandasana.com
403.229.2617

Editor: Patricia MacDonald

Associate Editors:
David Aldous
Suzette O'Byrne, Kinesiologist and Yoga Instructor
Margot Kitchen, Senior Iyengar Yoga Instructor
Janette Hurley, MD
Jennifer Steed, Yoga Instructor
Lorrie Maffey, Physiotherapist
George Huang, MD

International Standard Book Numbers:
ISBN 10: 0-939616-54-8
ISBN 13: 978-0-939616-54-1
Library of Congress Control Number: 2006920186
Printed in China

4   6   8   10   9   7   5

Book Design by WILLIAM JOSEPH

Disclaimer

The purpose of this book is to provide information for yoga instructors and enthusiasts on the subject of anatomy as it relates to asana. This book does not offer any medical advice to the reader and is not intended as a replacement for appropriate health care and treatment. For such advice, readers should consult their health care practitioners.

Countless people have helped me along the way in the process of writing and publishing this book. First and foremost, the **yoga instructors** and **students** whom I have taught over the years – you have taught me much about what it is to teach another; **Rob Walker** for initiating the very first Anatomy and Asana workshop at Yoga Studio South in Calgary; **Eoin Finn** for being the first yogi to upload my ezines to his website, **www.vancouveryoga.com**, which enabled more people to read the Anatomy and Asana ezines and become inspired to learn more about anatomy as it relates to asanas; **Ian Buchanon** for introducing Anatomy and Asana to his ashtanga yoga studio and supporting the production of this book by pre-buying in bulk; **Jennifer Steed** for being the bright shining light that I got to chat with each week at the studio and for supporting production of the book by pre-buying a large bulk order; **Lindsay McKechnie-Clague** for helping to spread the word through Vancouver; **Paulette Dennis** for her amazing drawings and willingness to do whatever it takes; **Suzette O'Byrne** for her cheerful editing and lovely way of being; **Dr. Jan Hurley, MD,** for her huge laugh and for editing section 1 for medical accuracy; **Lorrie Maffey, PT,** for her gentle critique of section 3; **Danielle Cregg, PT,** for being available to answer my questions; **Patricia MacDonald** for her grammatical and style editing, which brings true flow to my thoughts and words; **Patrick Anderson** and **Joe Bailey** for leading me to resources to help fill out my thoughts and ideas; **Annette Bossert** for reminding me to be connected; **Ink Tree Marketing** for helping with the small details and technicalities required to bring a manuscript to market; **WILLIAM JOSEPH** for their expertise in layout, design, and printing; and **Scott Paton** for helping with my website. Thanks **Suzette, Anne, Jodi, Marietta,** and **Cara,** who teach and work at Functional Synergy – your presence is inspiring. Saving best for last, my amazing husband, **Dave,** and my parents, **George** and **Nancy,** without whom I wouldn't have this incredible life.

acknowledgments

Relative to our physical existence, Prana or vital energy is a modification of the air element, primarily the oxygen we breathe that allows us to live. Yet, as air originates in ether or space, Prana arises in space and remains closely connected to it. Wherever we create space … energy or Prana must arise automatically.

— David Frawley

Space and Anatomy: Feeling the Flow

Yoga, at its essence, is a practice of energy – of creating space inside the body for prana to be cultivated, moved, and transformed for optimum health, well-being, connection, and ease. To be able to create space requires balance – balance of joint stability and mobility; balance of muscle contraction and relaxation; balance of movement between the limbs and the torso; and balance of the physical asana practice with the other seven limbs of yoga.

As balance is created and developed inside and through the body, by default, balance is created outside the body.

This book is intended as a tool for the exploration of balance – balance as a flowing, dynamic state, much like the ebb and flow of the tide.

I invite you to explore and feel.

The purpose of this book is to add to your exploration of the energy of yoga that is inside and outside of you. To give you tools to apply to your practice as a teacher and student of yoga.

Anatomy and Asana is based on relevant and current understanding of anatomical and kinesiological principles. I have used these principles both in my own practice and with my students, with very successful results. But please don't accept blindly what I have written on these pages. Please use the information to explore your own body in your practice. Feel what happens and let it become ingrained in you. I would love to know about your own "ah-has" as you experience the principles in your practice. Feel free to email them to me at ahhas@anatomyandasana.com.

How This Book Is Organized

Anatomy and Asana focuses on three themes:

- Understanding the movement components of anatomy as they relate to yoga asanas
- Understanding anatomy as it relates to asanas so that you can create space in your body to enable movement
- Understanding asanas as they relate to anatomy so that you can use movement to create space in your body

The book is divided into four sections. The first section dives under the skin into the internal world of our bodies. Section 2 takes us deeper into the language of anatomy and movement. Section 3 explores the principles of movement as they relate to yoga. Section 4 delves into applying the principles to the specific groups of yoga asanas – standing poses, back bends, forward bends, twists, and inversions. In each group, we'll look at where there is a tendency for injury and what we can do to instill space in our bodies and prevent injury from happening.

Sprinkled throughout the book are tips, for both teachers and students, to bring alive the concepts of anatomy in your practice of yoga.

Happy exploring,

Susi

introduction

contents

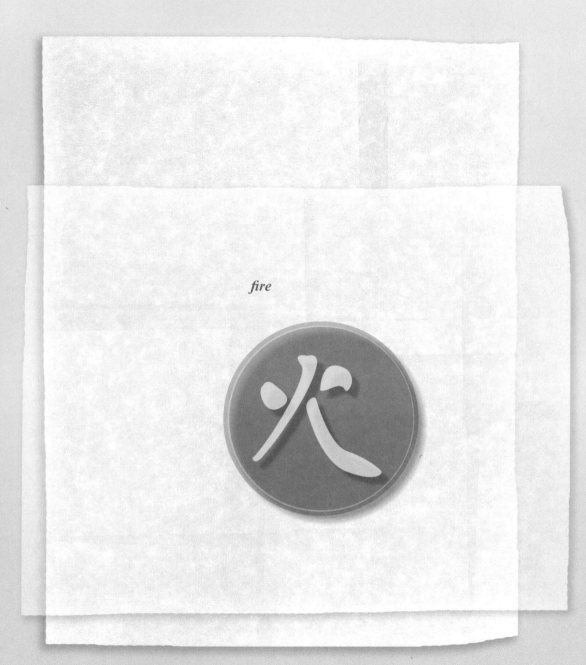

fire

Breathing in I calm the body and mind

Breathing out I smile

Dwelling in the present moment

I know this is the only moment

— *Thich Nhat Hanh*

the internal world

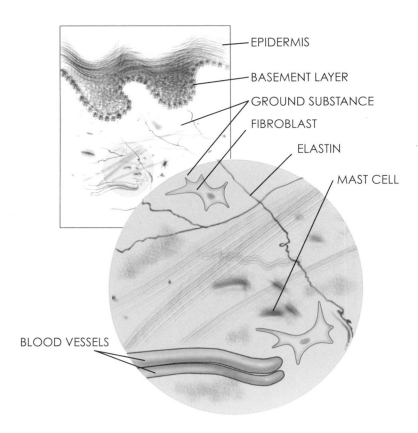

- EPIDERMIS
- BASEMENT LAYER
- GROUND SUBSTANCE
- FIBROBLAST
- ELASTIN
- MAST CELL
- BLOOD VESSELS

Fig 1-1 Beneath the skin

 Because of its vastness and influence on all parts of the body, connective tissue also has an influence on our practice of yoga.

the internal world

Let's delve beneath the skin and explore – explore the pieces that make up our physical bodies; the pieces that move us into and out of asanas; the pieces that nourish us; the pieces that give us lightness, ease, and flow.

Skin

The most visible organ of the body, skin provides three essential functions for our health, well-being, and practice of yoga.

- It covers organs and tissues and protects them from impact and infection.
- It regulates body temperature.
- It contains receptors that distinguish sensations such as touch, pressure, vibration, pain, and temperature change.

Connective Tissue

If I were to cut myself open, I would find connective tissue directly underneath the layer of surface skin *(fig 1-1)*. If I were to cut open a blood vessel, I would find connective tissue directly inside. I would also find connective tissue surrounding the elements of muscle and creating the structure of bones, tendons, ligaments, and fascia. In all, connective tissue is vast. It is found throughout the body in various forms, conducting various functions, including the following:

- Creating the structural framework of the body
- Transporting fluids from one region of the body to another
- Protecting organs
- Supporting, surrounding, and interconnecting neighbouring tissues and structures
- Storing energy reserves
- Defending the body from invading micro-organisms[1]

Because of its vastness and influence on all parts of the body, connective tissue also has an influence on our practice of yoga. Let's delve deeper into its structure and function.

There are three categories of connective tissue:

- Connective tissue proper, which includes fat, tendons, ligaments, and fascia
- Supporting connective tissue, which includes cartilage and bone
- Fluid connective tissue, which includes blood and lymph

Connective Tissue Proper: Tendons, Ligaments, and Fascia

Connective tissue proper has a few different forms depending on where it is located in the body. It can occur in the form of tightly aligned fibers arranged like a rope; or as a multidirectional array of fibers arranged as a tough but far-reaching network; or as a wavy, highly flexible fiber that interconnects vertebrae. Although it has a few different forms, all connective tissue proper is created by the same cells, called fibroblasts.

Fibroblasts are responsible for the production and maintenance of the fibers that create connective tissue proper. To explore how fibroblasts work, imagine a spider spinning a web of three distinct and resilient fibers:

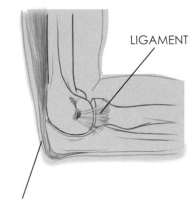

LIGAMENT

TENDON OF TRICEPS BRACHII
Fig 1-2

1

Collagen is the most common fiber. It consists of strong strands of fibers that when wound together are strong and flexible, like a piece of rope when it is stretched from end to end. You will find collagen as the primary component in tendons, ligaments, and fascia.

2

Reticular fibers are thinner than collagen yet are still tough and flexible. Rather than being aligned like collagen fibers, reticular fibers form a network. This network style of organization enables them to resist forces from a multitude of directions, which is particularly useful when we move into inversions.

Even when we are upside down, the relative position of our organs, nerves, and blood vessels doesn't change. This is due, in part, to the networking arrangement of the reticular fibers.

3

Elastic fibers are the rarest of the three fibers. These branching, wavy fibers are able to stretch up to 150% of their original resting length and recoil with ease. They can be found in the ligaments between each of the vertebrae. Since they stabilize the position of the vertebrae and cushion the shock, elastic fibers are useful when we land after jumping into asanas or when we move into yoga asanas that require the spine to bend or twist.

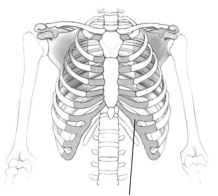

COSTAL CARTILAGE
Fig 1-3

Examples of connective tissue proper in action

Tendons are bands of collagen fibers that act as the bridge between muscle and bone. Strong and fibrous, tendons provide a solid foundation for leveraging the body into movement (fig 1-2).

Yoga students sometimes push themselves too hard and tear the hamstring tendon while in Adho Mukha Svanasana (Downward Facing Dog). Considering that a bone is more easily broken than a tendon is torn, you can imagine how strong a force is required for someone to tear her hamstring tendon.

Ligaments are also strong fibrous bands of collagen. Connecting bone to bone, ligaments provide firm support to joints so that bones do not move out of alignment.

Fascia creates the internal framework of the body by connecting, separating, attaching, stabilizing, and enclosing muscles and other internal organs. (More on fascia on page 14.)

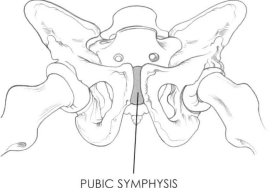

PUBIC SYMPHYSIS
Fig 1-4

Notice that the stiffest tree is most easily cracked, while the bamboo or willow survives by bending with the wind.

Supporting Connective Tissue: Cartilage and Bone

As the second division of connective tissue, supporting connective tissue offers a strong structural and supportive framework in the form of cartilage and bone.

The primary difference between supporting connective tissue and connective tissue proper is the density of fibers. In supporting connective tissue, the fibers are more densely packed and in some cases contain calcium salts, which provide rigidity and strength.

Cartilage provides support, reduces friction between bony surfaces, reduces compression, absorbs shock, and prevents bone-on-bone contact.[2] Depending on where it is located in the body, it is mostly composed of collagen fibers or elastic fibers. There are three types of cartilage. Hyaline cartilage, which is composed of tightly packed collagen fibers, creates the costal cartilage *(fig 1-3)* between the ribs and the sternum as well as the articular cartilage *(fig 1-5)* lining the surface of the knee and elbow. Elastic cartilage, which as its name implies is composed mostly of elastic fibers, can be found in the outer flap of the ear and in the epiglottis. Fibrocartilage is the toughest and most durable of the three. It is composed of tightly woven collagen fibers that make up the cartilage at the pubic symphysis *(fig 1-4)*, form the spinal discs between the vertebrae, and interweave with some joints and tendons.

Bone is, by some definitions, tougher and more durable than cartilage. Collagen fibers make up one third of bone, while the remaining two thirds is a combination of calcium salts. The combination of the collagen fibers and calcium salts makes bone quite strong, flexible, and resistant to breaking.

Fluid Connective Tissue: Blood and Lymph

While tendons, ligaments, and fascia are composed of fibers in sheets or bands, blood and lymph are connective tissues that are more watery-like. Under normal conditions, fluid connective tissue doesn't form fibers like those found in cartilage, bone, tendons, or ligaments. (More on blood and lymph on pages 16–17.)

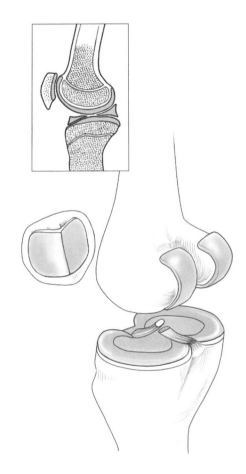

Fig 1-5 Articular cartilage

Muscles

As we delve deeper into the body, beneath the connective tissue muscle will be found *(fig 1-6)*. Muscle provides the force behind movement – and not just movement of our bones. It is also the force behind:

- the movement of blood and lymph,
- the expansion and contraction of the lungs, and
- the movement of solids and fluids through the digestive tract.

There are three different types of muscle in our body: smooth muscle, cardiac muscle, and skeletal muscle. Smooth muscle lines all of the organs, the blood vessels, and the digestive tract. Cardiac muscle resides in the heart, where its structure specifically contributes to pushing blood through the arteries and veins. Skeletal muscle is the vehicle for direct movement of the bones. Since this book is specific to movement and yoga asanas, the focus will be on skeletal muscle.

Skeletal Muscle

In addition to moving our bones into and out of yoga asanas, skeletal muscle has three other duties:

1. Skeletal muscle maintains our posture. While our arms and legs move from Tadasana (Mountain Pose) into Vrksasana (Tree Pose), our heads and necks stay in the same position. Without constant contraction of the skeletal muscles, our heads would not stay upright.

2. Skeletal muscle supports our internal organs. All of the internal organs are supported by skeletal muscle, so that when we are in Uttanasana (Standing Forward Bend) or in Adho Mukha Vrksasana (Handstand), our internal organs remain in the same relative position.

3. Skeletal muscle encircles our orifices, including the anus, vagina, and urethra. We use these muscles to access mula bandha deep in the pelvis (anal muscles release while the muscles of the vagina [for women] and urethra contract).

Skeletal muscle is composed of layers and layers of fibers. Inside of one fiber are hundreds and thousands of myofibrils. Inside each myofibril are bundles of myofilaments, which are protein filaments. These protein filaments, called actin and myosin, are organized in units called sarcomeres. It is here at the actin and myosin where the force of muscle is created. (For more on muscle contraction and movement, read nerve–muscle communication on page 12.)

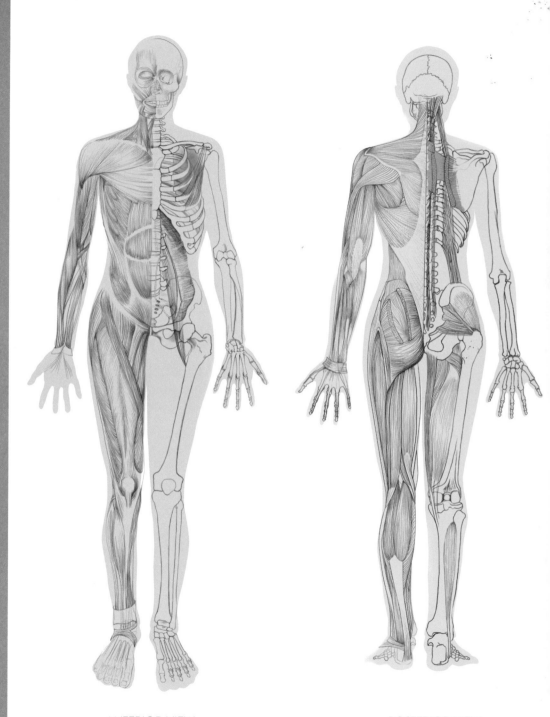

ANTERIOR VIEW   POSTERIOR VIEW

Fig 1-6 Skeletal muscle

The Skeleton and Its Bones

As you delve deeper, beneath the muscle you will discover the bones that make up the skeleton *(fig 1-7)*. The skeleton provides:

- a structural framework for our bodies,
- the attachment site for tendons,
- support and protection for internal organs, and
- calcium and mineral storage,
- red blood cell production.

As it relates to yoga, the skeleton is not typically the first image that comes to mind when we think of anatomy and asanas. Rather, we tend to think of bones as the attachment site for tendons and ligaments or as a concept of alignment – "stack your bones."

So let's take one step further and explore how bones connect and move

Joints: Connecting Bones, Creating Movement

While we depend on our muscles to create force, thereby allowing our bones to move from one asana into the next, our joints are the parts that contribute to fluidity of movement. Without joints we would be nothing more than statues.

Why is this so?

Our bones are rigid pieces. It is impossible to bend them as we bend wood when creating a spiral staircase. Instead, we rely on joint movement to help us bend, twist, arch, and extend.

Joints are the connecting points between two bones. Some are small, some are large. Some move a lot, some move very little.

The following is a list of joints based on the amount of movement available and some examples in the body where you will find this type of joint. As you read the table, consider how the joint movement available in that part of your body supports your physical asanas.[3]

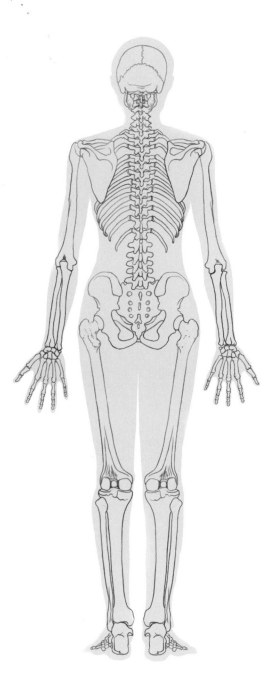

Fig 1-7 Posterior view of the skeleton

Amount of Movement	Description	Example	
Very, very minute movement	The bones of these joints sit very close together or even interlock; they are bound together by dense connective tissue	The bones of the skull	
A wee bit of movement	The bones of these joints sit a little farther apart; they are connected by ligaments or cartilage	The pubic symphysis and the intervertebral discs; the joint between the tibia and fibula at its distal end – close to the ankle	
Free and easy movement	The bones of these joints do not touch each other (under normal circumstances) because they are separated by articular cartilage, which reduces friction and provides shock absorption	The elbow, ankle, ribs, wrist, shoulder, and hip	

Joints and Our Western Culture

In our Western culture, we are beginning to lose some of the functioning of our larger joints, such as the traditionally healthy joints at the shoulders and hips. As a result our smaller joints – our elbows, wrists, knees, ankles, and vertebrae – must take on a larger load. To maintain and improve our functioning, it is important to accentuate the movement at these larger joints so that we can take the pressure off the smaller ones.

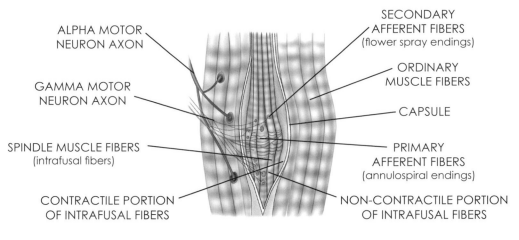

ALPHA MOTOR NEURON AXON

GAMMA MOTOR NEURON AXON

SPINDLE MUSCLE FIBERS (intrafusal fibers)

CONTRACTILE PORTION OF INTRAFUSAL FIBERS

SECONDARY AFFERENT FIBERS (flower spray endings)

ORDINARY MUSCLE FIBERS

CAPSULE

PRIMARY AFFERENT FIBERS (annulospiral endings)

NON-CONTRACTILE PORTION OF INTRAFUSAL FIBERS

Fig 1-8 Sensors deep inside the muscle

Nerves

Nerves supply the electrical connection from the brain and spinal cord to every part of the body. Specific to muscle, nerves provide and receive feedback about how much a muscle has moved, the force needed to move it (or stop it from moving), and when to shift from contraction to relaxation.

Nerve–Muscle Communication: Nerve Sensors Inside the Muscle

In order for the muscle fibers to know what to do and how much to do it, they rely on "sensors." These sensors (fig 1-8) lie deep inside the muscle and provide information such as how much to contract and how much to relax. They gauge how quickly or how far the muscle is moving and give feedback (through the nervous system) to the muscle fibers, telling them to continue to contract, continue to relax, stop contracting, or stop relaxing.

Two of these sensors are the muscle spindle and Golgi tendon organ.

Muscle spindles run parallel to the muscle fibers and sense how far and how fast the fibers are stretching. If the muscle is stretching too far or too fast, the muscle spindle will be activated, creating a "stretch reflex." This will cause the stretched muscle to automatically contract, preventing possible damage from overstretching.

In yoga asanas, if you move into your postures too quickly or too far, your muscle spindles will respond by causing your muscles to contract forcefully, preventing the stretch from happening. The degree to which your muscle spindles activate the stretch reflex depends on how quickly you are moving. The faster you go, the stronger the reflex, and the stronger the ensuing contraction.

Sometimes instructors may use over-zealous adjustments on students. These overzealous adjustments can actually cause the students' muscles to contract more than release. One of the reasons lies in the stretch reflex. If the teacher moves a student's body too fast or too far, the muscle spindles' stretch reflex will be triggered. Instead of further release through the muscle, the muscle resists by contracting.

While the muscle spindles lie parallel to the muscle fibers, the Golgi tendon organs reside mostly at either end of the muscle near the junction of the muscle and tendon. Golgi tendon organs are primarily sensitive to the amount of tension in the muscle, so when there is an increase of tension (contraction), they discharge, causing the muscle to relax.

How do the muscle spindles and Golgi tendon organs differ?

The muscle spindles are sensitive to both how fast and how far the muscle stretches. If you stretch too fast or too far, they will engage the stretch reflex, causing the muscle to contract. The Golgi tendon organs, on the other hand, are more sensitive to contraction. So if there is too much tension, the Golgi tendon organs will discharge, causing the muscle to relax.

How do I avoid triggering the stretch reflex?

Move with your breath, move with ease, move at your own pace, be thoughtful and conscious – those time-honoured words have science behind them. If you are moving with your steady and easy breath, if you are moving with ease and at your own pace, you are moving at a speed that won't trigger the stretch reflex. The result is that you will be able to settle into the pose completely and experience a safe yet deep release.

How does the Golgi tendon organ work in the world beyond the textbook?

In the sport, fitness, and rehabilitation world, a stretching technique utilizes the function of the Golgi tendon organ to create greater flexibility. This kind of stretching is called PNF (proprioceptive neuromuscular facilitation), or contract–relax stretching. It is possible to use this type of stretching in yoga asanas.

Here is an example:

Imagine lying on your back in a basic Supta Padangusthasana (Supine Hamstring Stretch). A partner is helping you stretch by placing his or her hand on your foot and taking your leg (that is being stretched) to your almost maximum hamstring stretch. At that point, you press your foot against your partner's hand, causing your hamstrings to contract (hold this for 10 seconds), and then relax the leg. Typically, your leg will now stretch further. Studies suggest that the 10-second contraction of the hamstring muscles discharges the Golgi tendon organ, which in turn relaxes the muscles, overrides the stretch reflex, and causes a greater stretch.

How does PNF stretching differ from static stretching?

PNF stretching is quite different from static stretching, since static stretching is just that – static. Moving back to Supta Padangusthasana, in a static stretch version of this asana, you hold your leg with your hands or a strap, allowing the stretch to occur as it may. Typically, the longer you stay in the stretch, the more your muscles will release.

Which one is better?

That is up to the scientists to debate and for you to experience and decide for yourself. Sometimes PNF can lead to injury because the person overcontracts his muscles, or his partner overstretches the muscles, leading to muscle tearing. Other times, when performed correctly, PNF can be a valuable method of increasing flexibility.

On the other hand, static stretching requires a lot of focus and patience, but it is safe and you know it works.

The Organizational Network: Fascia

I have often joked that, as humans, we are walking "skin bags" filled with different parts – bones, muscles, tendons, ligaments, organs, nerves, vessels, and a brain. Many people are happy just knowing that this sac stays intact, its contents contained.

Others, such as yogi anatomists, are more interested in how it is organized, how it works, and how we can help it function better.

One of the keys to this deeper understanding is fascia. In many texts, fascia is described as a body envelope, or sac, permeating through and around every nook of the body. It surrounds nerve fibers, surrounds and bundles muscle fibers, and lines organs and vessels. It is the element that gives contour and structure to the body, linking the pieces together into segments, segments together into systems. In essence, fascia connects all of our parts and organizes them into a vibrant whole.

The structure, look, and feel of fascia vary depending on what it is enveloping or lining. It varies from the thin, glossy, slick covering that surrounds bone to a thicker gristle-like, white covering that wraps around muscle.

Structure and Functions of Fascia

Fascia was first introduced on page 8 as connective tissue proper, which is composed primarily of collagen fibers. In this section, let's take a closer look at fascia. There are three levels of fascia:

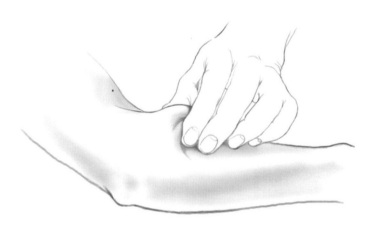

Fig 1-9 In pinching the skin, you are also pinching superficial fascia.

Moving from Bhujangasana (Cobra Pose) into Adho Mukha Svanasana (Downward Facing Dog), your muscles are contracting and releasing. As they contract and release, they are not getting caught in the skin that lies above. This is due to the superficial fascia.

1

Superficial

Superficial fascia resides just underneath the skin. To explore your superficial fascia, take a moment and pinch your skin *(fig 1-9)*, but not your muscle. In that pinch of skin, you are also pinching superficial fascia. The role of superficial fascia is to provide insulation and padding while letting the skin and the underlying structures, such as muscles, move independently of each other.

2

Deep

Deep fascia is denser than superficial or subserous fascia, and because of the arrangement of collagen fibers, offers the greatest resiliency of the three types of fascia. In deep fascia, the collagen fibers are arranged in layers. Within one layer, the fibers are aligned in one direction; between layers, the direction of fibers changes slightly. These qualities of fiber alignment within layers and between layers help the deep fascia resist forces applied from many different directions, such as when we move our bodies into Trikonasana (Triangle Pose).

Deep fascia creates a strong fibrous network tying structural elements together. It is this type of fascia that encloses muscle, blends into the fibers that create tendons, and then intermingles with those fibers that make up the fascia surrounding bone.

3

Subserous

Subserous fascia lies between the deep fascia and the lining of body cavities. This prevents the movements of muscles or organs from deforming or interfering with this sensitive lining.

The Role of Yoga and Fascia

Yoga is a brilliant form of movement that nourishes and rejuvenates the functioning of fascia. The asanas engage and release all angles of the body; inspire movement in different directions; and encourage relaxation, effortless effort, and easy breathing – all components necessary for properly functioning fascia.

So next time you hug your arm around your leg as you gently deepen into Marichyasana (Pose Dedicated to the Sage Marichi), flow from Tadasana to Uttanasana (Mountain Pose to Standing Forward Bend), settle into Virabhadrasana 2 (Warrior 2 Pose), or release into any of your favourite back bends, know that beneath the skin the organizing structure of fascia is loving it.

How Fascia Organizes Muscle:
Peeling the Orange

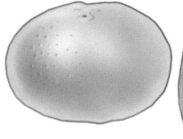
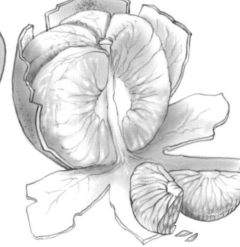

The organizational relationship between muscle and fascia is similar to that of an orange *(fig 1-10)*: a broad sheet of fascia encases the whole fruit, deeper layers of fascia separate the orange into "wedges" (the portions you eat after peeling), and finally, a thin coating of tissue surrounds each tiny bud of fruit. Applying this analogy to muscle, a layer of fascia encases the muscle as a whole, a deeper layer wraps the long muscle fibers into bundles, and finally, each microscopic muscle fiber is bound in fascia. Unlike an orange, a muscle's layers of connective tissue merge at either end of the muscle to form a strong tendon. The tendon attaches the muscle to bone.[4]

Fig 1-10

Understanding shatters old knowledge to make room for the new that accords with reality.

— *Thich Nhat Hanh*

Circulation

Whether your yoga practice is a flow style of yoga or whether it is more static, you will feel to some degree the movement of fluid through your body. It may be through feeling the pulse of blood through your blood vessels, or it may be through hearing the beating of your heart as you become more and more quiet in your practice.

Fluid flows through the body in the form of blood or lymph. Blood flows through the cardiovascular system (fig 1-11), while lymph flows through the lymphatic system (fig 1-12) Together, blood and lymph transport and exchange nutrients, metabolic waste products, and hormones necessary for energy.

Blood Vessels

Blood vessels carry blood from the heart to the lungs, from the heart to the rest of the body, and from the body back to the heart. In this way, they operate as a two-way return system. Blood flows both away from and toward its primary pump, the heart.

Blood vessels are divided into three distinct vessels called arteries, veins, and capillaries.

As blood is pumped from the heart toward the limbs of the body, it moves through a series of arteries ranging in size and diameter. Initially, blood enters elastic arteries, which handle large volumes of blood. Elastic arteries include the pulmonary, common carotid, subclavian, and common iliac arteries. These elastic arteries bring the blood to muscular arteries. Muscular arteries distribute blood to skeletal muscle and internal organs. These arteries are thinner than the elastic arteries and include the femoral arteries in the thighs, the external carotid arteries in the neck, and the brachial arteries in the arms. From the muscular arteries, blood flows into arterioles. Arterioles are the smallest in the group of arteries and control the blood flow between the larger arteries and the capillaries.

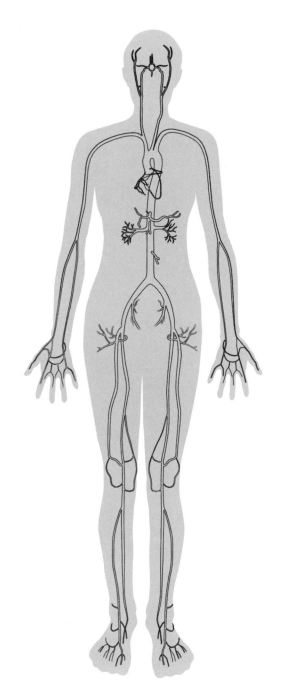

Fig 1-11 Cardiovascular system

Yoga and Blood Flow

Blood flow can be impeded by stress. In the cardiovascular system, the body responds to stress by constricting the smaller blood vessels – the arterioles, capillaries, and venules. Since the arterioles, capillaries, and venules are located in the areas farthest from the heart, constricted blood flow due to stress is experienced as cold hands and feet. The rhythmic movement of a yoga asana practice (whether vinyasa, static, or restorative) regulates breathing and eases stress and tension. This helps dissipate the experience of stress, improving the blood flow to the hands and the feet.

Capillaries are the smallest of the blood vessels. They are necessary for exchange of nutrients between the blood vessels and adjacent parts of the body.

From the capillaries, blood returns to the heart through the system of veins. It travels first through venules, the smallest of the veins, which sometimes look like an expanded series of capillaries. From the venules, blood moves into medium sized veins. Once through the medium sized veins, blood enters the large veins and then into the heart. In both the venules and medium sized veins, the blood pressure is too low to move effectively against gravity. To help blood in its travels back to the heart, a series of venous valves are designed to prevent backflow. Any pressure on the valve will help it push the blood toward the heart.

Lymphatic Vessels

Lymphatic vessels are part of the larger lymphatic system *(fig 1-12)*, which networks together the lymphatic vessels, lymph nodes, lymphoid organs, spleen, thymus, and tonsils. These tissues and organs work to destroy bacteria and maintain the volume of blood in the bloodstream. The lymphatic system is a one-way system – fluid is received then transported to the bloodstream. A return mechanism, like that for the blood vessels, does not exist.

Like the blood vessels, lymphatic vessels vary in size. The smallest lymphatic vessels are the lymphatic capillaries. Lymphatic capillaries are located in almost every tissue in the body. From the capillaries, lymph travels into larger vessels called lymphatic trunks and then into lymphatic ducts. Lymphatic ducts empty the lymph into the blood system.

Lymphatic trunks and ducts are similar to veins in that they require one-way valves to help push along the fluid. The one-way valves make the lymphatic ducts bulge out slightly, making this system look like a string of beads.

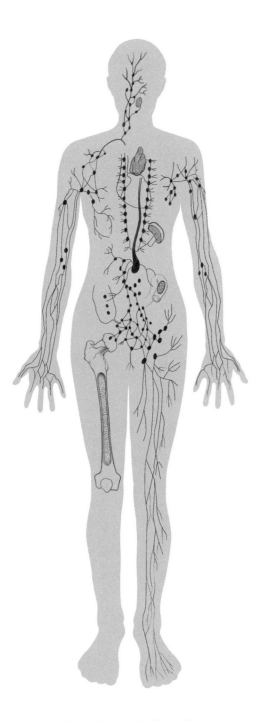

Fig 1-12 Lymphatic system

Yoga and Lymphatic Flow

In addition to the one-way valves that help push the lymph through the vessels, lymphatic flow also relies on skeletal muscle contractions and breathing. Muscle contractions in the arms and legs compress the lymphatic vessels and squeeze the lymph toward the trunk.

A similar situation occurs in breathing. With an inhalation, pressure decreases in the thoracic cavity, and the lymph is pulled from the smaller lymphatic vessels into the larger lymphatic ducts.

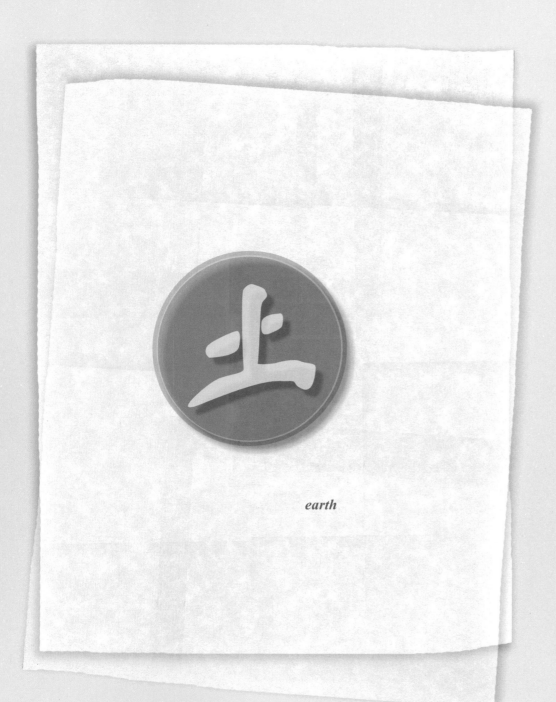

earth

As you go on breathing in this frame of mind, with these associations, alternating between movement and stillness, it is important that the focus of your mind does not shift. Let the true breath come and go, a subtle continuum on the brink of existence. Tune the breathing until you get breath without breathing; become one with it, and then the spirit can be solidified and the elixir can be made.

— *Chang San-Feng*

language of anatomy

language of anatomy

Exploring and experiencing anatomy is similar to exploring and experiencing yoga asanas. Both are navigated with their own distinct languages.

In yoga, the language is one of cueing. Cueing communicates how to feel the asana, where to place your feet, how to feel your breath, and how to relax while strengthening. Without it, a yoga practitioner would be left mindless, unsure of which direction her body should be going.

Anatomy is the same. With multiple systems and thousands of bodily bits and pieces, the language of anatomy provides a system of communication to enable professionals from all aspects of health and well-being to communicate accurately.

When first learning anatomy, this language may be overwhelming. As you stick with it, your understanding of anatomy and how it relates to yoga asanas will only improve.

Anatomical Landmarks

The anatomical landmarks are important as they pertain to anatomy and asanas. As you learn them, you will understand more about how the muscles get their names.

Anatomical Position and Anatomical Direction

Anatomical descriptions are always expressed in relation to the basic anatomical position. The anatomical position is very similar to Tadasana (Mountain Pose) or Savasana (Corpse Pose). In fig 2-1 on page 20, the drawings of each of the planes show the person in anatomical position. By understanding anatomical position, you will understand the relationship of any part of the body to any other part of the body.

Anatomical Direction and Human Anatomy: Terms to Describe the Body's Relationship to Anatomical Position		
Superior	Nearer to the head	The eyes are superior to the chin
Inferior	Nearer to the feet	The knee is inferior to the hip
Lateral	Away from the center longitudinal line of the body	The lateral edge of the foot is the outside edge
Medial	Toward the center longitudinal line of the body	The big toe is on the medial side of the foot
Anterior (Ventral)	Nearer to the front or on the front	The navel is on the anterior surface of the torso
Posterior (Dorsal)	Nearer to the back or on the back	The scapulae, or shoulder blades, are on the posterior surface of the torso

Terms to Describe Body Parts in Relation to Their Position		
Distal	Farther from the trunk	The hand is distal to the elbow
Proximal	Nearer to the trunk	The shoulder is proximal to the elbow
Deep	Farther from the surface	The organs are deep to the skin
Superficial	Nearer to or at the surface	The skin is superficial to the organs
Ipsilateral	On the same side of the body	The right shoulder and right hip are ipsilateral
Contralateral	On the opposite side of the body	The right shoulder and left hip are contralateral

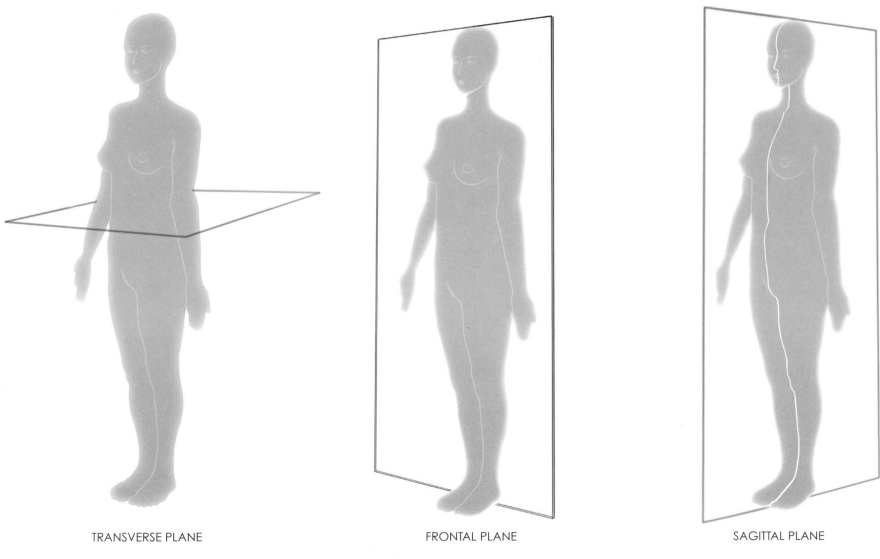

TRANSVERSE PLANE   FRONTAL PLANE   SAGITTAL PLANE

Fig 2-1 The planes of the body

Planes of the Body

When describing movement, it becomes easier to describe it according to the anatomical planes. Anatomical planes are imaginary lines that run through the body. There are three anatomical planes: transverse, frontal, and sagittal.

The transverse plane is perpendicular to the longitudinal, or central, axis of the body. It splits the body into superior and inferior sections. The frontal plane extends from side to side, dividing the body into anterior and posterior sections. The sagittal plane runs from anterior to posterior and divides the body into right and left.

Movements of the Body

All movement occurs at the joints by way of muscles releasing or contracting. Related to yoga asanas, muscles release or contract to move bones at their joints. Therefore, to understand muscle action and muscle function, it is important to understand joint movement relative to the anatomical position.

Flexion

Flexion moves in the sagittal plane. Flexion causes the joint angle to become smaller. Hip flexion reduces the angle of the hip joint.

Extension

Extension moves in the sagittal plane. Extension causes the joint angle to become greater. Hip extension increases the angle of the hip joint.

Abduction

Abduction moves in the frontal plane, side to side. Abduction is a position or motion that moves a segment away from the midline of the body.

Adduction

Adduction moves in the frontal plane, side to side. Adduction is a position or motion that moves a segment toward the midline of the body.

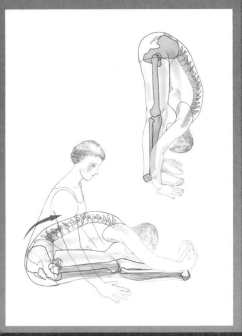
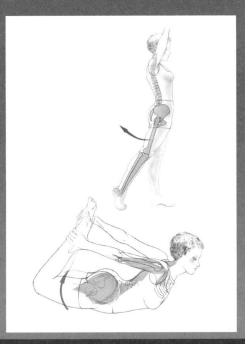
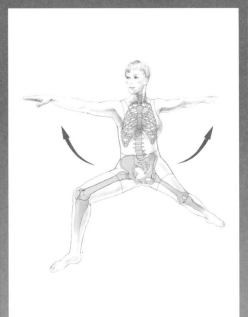
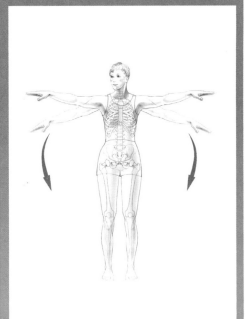

Without full awareness of breathing, there can be no development of meditative stability and understanding.

— Thich Nhat Hanh

Rotation	External (Lateral) Rotation	Internal (Medial) Rotation	Supination	Pronation
Rotation moves in the transverse plane. Rotation of the spine occurs in twists.	External (lateral) rotation occurs in the transverse plane away from the midline of the body. In standing, the femur at the hip joint moves in external rotation when it rolls outward.	Internal (medial) rotation occurs in the transverse plane toward the midline of the body. In standing, the femur at the hip joint moves in internal rotation when it rolls inward.	Supination is a form of external rotation of the forearm or foot.	Pronation is a form of internal rotation of the forearm or foot. The forearms are pronated in Pincha Mayurasana (Forearm Stand).

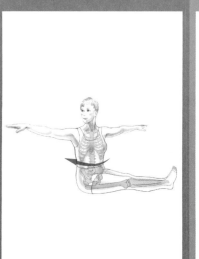

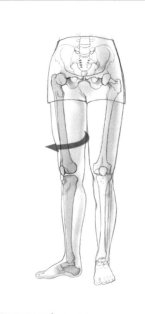

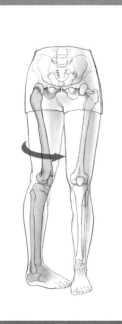

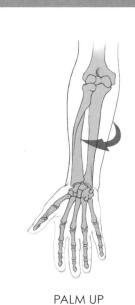

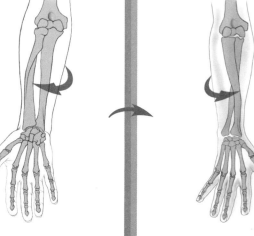

PALM UP

PALM DOWN

Shoulder, Scapulae, and Torso Movements

Horizontal Flexion

Horizontal flexion occurs when the arm is in 90 degrees of abduction, or directly in line with the shoulder joint. The movement is in the transverse plane toward the center line of the body.

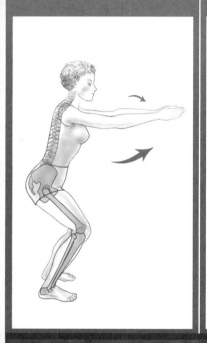

Horizontal Extension

Horizontal extension occurs when the arm is in 90 degrees of abduction, or directly in line with the shoulder joint. The movement is in the transverse plane, away from the center line of the body.

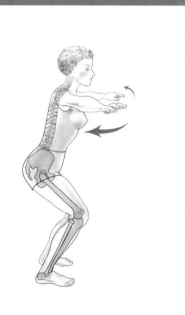

Retraction

Retraction occurs at the scapulae and brings the scapulae toward the spine. We typically retract our scapulae in back bends.

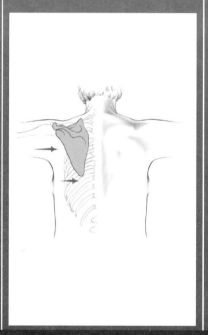

Protraction

Protraction occurs at the scapulae and brings the scapulae away from the spine. Protraction occurs in Chaturanga Dandasana (Four-Limbed Staff Pose).

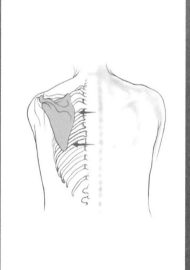

Elevation

Elevation occurs at the scapulae, bringing them up toward the ears. We don't typically elevate the scapulae in yoga asanas.

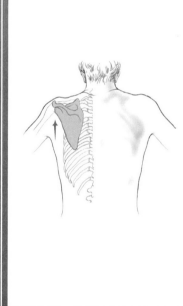

Special Movements

Dorsiflexion and plantar flexion defy the rules of joint movement according to planes *(fig 2-2)*. It is accepted that when the superior, or dorsal, surface of the foot moves toward the tibia, the movement is dorsiflexion. When the plantar surface, or sole, of the foot moves toward the floor, the movement is plantar flexion.

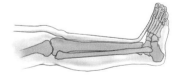 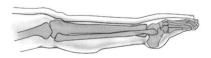

DORSIFLEXION   PLANTAR FLEXION

Fig 2-2 Dorsiflexion and Plantar Flexion

(Shoulder, Scapulae, and Torso Movements continued)

Depression

Depression occurs at the scapulae, moving them down the back of the body. We depress our shoulder blades in most yoga asanas, such as Bhujangasana (Cobra Pose).

Lateral Flexion

Lateral flexion occurs in the torso and looks like a side bend.

Going Deeper: The Relationships between Muscles

So far, the language has focused on anatomical position, planes of the body, and movements of the body as they relate to the anatomical position and the planes. This section takes that understanding a little deeper by exploring the relationship between muscles.

As mentioned earlier, muscles must contract or release to move a bone at its joint. But there is more to it than that. To truly move a bone at its joint, three things must occur. A set (or two sets) of muscles must contract, another set must release, and a third set must stabilize.[1]

Let's take a look:

Prime Movers
Prime movers are also known as the agonist muscles. They are the group of muscles that is predominantly contracting to cause the movement to occur.

Synergists
Synergists are buddies of the prime movers. They help the prime movers carry out the motion. If the prime movers are not functioning properly, the synergists may compensate to ensure the movement occurs.

Antagonists
Antagonists perform motion in the opposite direction of the agonist muscles. They are stretched passively during the movement and under normal circumstances do not affect the range of motion. However, if the antagonist muscles are tight or shortened, they may influence the movement.

Stabilizers
Stabilizers do not perform movement but rather fix the necessary part of the body so that movement can occur. The better the stabilizers are able to do their job, the more easily the movement will occur and the more fluid the pose.

Example: Bhujangasana (Cobra Pose) without using hands – Pure spinal extension

Prime mover: Erector spinae
Synergists: Semispinalis, interspinalis, quadratus lumborum
Antagonists: Various muscles, including the rectus abdominis
Stabilizers: Hamstrings, gluteus maximus, hip adductors, transversus abdominis

When movement is limited, what is happening?

When movement is limited, one or more of the following are occurring:

- The prime mover and its synergists are weak and unable to contract enough to bring the joint through its full range of motion.
- The antagonists are too shortened or tight, which prevents the prime mover from carrying out the movement.
- The stabilizers are not creating a supportive base from which to move.
- An anatomical change in the joint – such as arthritis – prevents full movement.
- Pain limits range of motion.

24   Anatomy and Asana: Preventing Yoga Injuries

Mechanics of Muscle Contraction

One of the beauties of yoga is the pureness of movement it creates. In many cases, no equipment is required – just body, mind, and mat. We breathe and our muscles contract and release. We move into forward bends, back bends, standing poses, twists, and inversions, and our muscles contract and release. No matter how dynamic, static, or restorative your particular practice, the contracting and releasing of muscles can truly become a dance.

We know the feeling of contraction and release. We know the feeling of lengthening and stretching. Many of us have heard and experienced the cue "Breathe through muscle," knowing that this will help our muscles relax. But what is the anatomical basis for what we are feeling and for the cues we are hearing?

Muscle Contraction

Muscles contract in a few different ways to create the action we are intending. The following is a description of the terminology we use to describe muscle contraction.

Isometric contraction: Isometric contractions are static contractions, producing no noticeable change in the angle of the joint. For example, when we are standing in Tadasana (Mountain Pose), there is no noticeable change in any of our joint angles. Our key postural muscles respon-

sible for keeping us in Tadasana are contracting isometrically. These are also the type of contractions we use when we stay in an asana for an extended period of time, without changing our body position. As soon as we move a limb, the muscles that moved that limb are no longer contracting isometrically.

Concentric contraction: Concentric contractions cause movement against gravity. They are a shortening contraction of the muscle. For example, when we are standing in Tadasana and we raise our arms and hands forward and toward our ears overhead, the anterior deltoid and biceps brachii muscles contract concentrically.

Eccentric contraction: Eccentric contractions slow down movement with gravity. They create lengthening contraction of a muscle. (Keep in mind that this term *lengthening* is not the same as our common yoga term *lengthening*.) From the previous example, if we lower our arms from overhead back to our sides, by coming forward and down, the biceps brachii and anterior deltoid contract eccentrically to keep the movement controlled so our arms don't fall down too fast.

A tip to remember: Whenever you are moving against gravity, you are creating a concentric contraction. Whenever you are moving with gravity, you are creating an eccentric contraction.

Here are more examples of different types of muscle contraction:

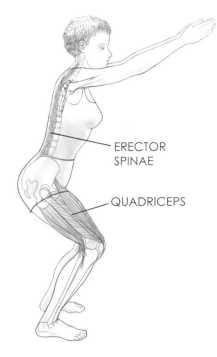

ERECTOR SPINAE

QUADRICEPS

Fig 2-3 Utkatasana

Focus on the Quadriceps Muscles Moving from Tadasana (Mountain Pose) into Utkatasana (Fierce/Powerful Pose) and Back to Tadasana	
Tadasana	Isometric contraction of the quadriceps
Into Utkatasana	Eccentric contraction of the quadriceps
Stay in Utkatasana	Isometric contraction of the quadriceps
Back to Tadasana	Concentric contraction of the quadriceps

(Keep in mind that more muscles are involved in this motion; for the sake of an example, we are focusing on the quadriceps.)

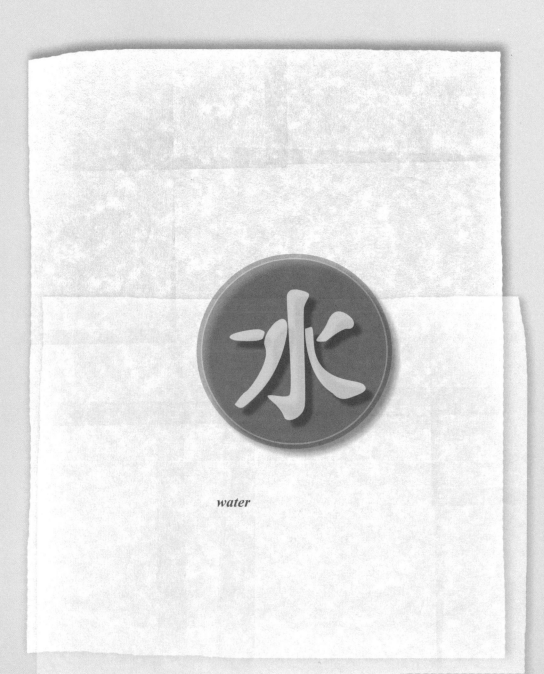

water

When the mind

settles on the mountain,

it becomes the mountain.

— *Thich Nhat Hanh*

principles

principles

Principles of Physiology Associated with Yoga Asanas

In exercise physiology, six foundational principles are key to health and well-being as they pertain to exercise. You will see that these principles are as applicable to asana practice as they are to traditional forms of exercise.

1

Principle of Individual Differences

Because every body and every mind are different, each person's response to a yoga asana practice will be different. The length of time between sessions will depend on the circumstances of each individual yogini – how new she is to yoga, her ability to connect brain and body, her level of fatigue, her level of stress, the amount of injury or scar tissue that exists in her body, and her age are just a few factors. These factors will also influence the style of yoga that a particular yogini is best suited for.

2

Principle of Overload

According to this principle, a yogi needs to apply a greater than normal stress on his body in order to adapt, change, and strengthen. You can do this for yourself by increasing the length of time you hold an asana or by increasing the complexity of the asana you are practicing. If you want to maintain the practice at its current level, then continue your practice as is.

3

Principle of Progression

This principle implies that there is an optimal level of overload for each of us. It is as important to rest and recover as it is to increase the complexity of or time in an asana. If a yogini increases the complexity of an asana or time in an asana too quickly, there is a greater chance for injury and a reduced chance for improvement. If the principle of progression is not followed, it is possible to overtrain. You know that you are overtraining in your yoga asana practice if you feel tired or dehydrated, experience ongoing muscular pain or insomnia, and are unable to relax.

Breathing control
gives man
strength,
vitality,
inspiration,
and magic powers.

— *Chuang Tzu*

A word of caution: As a teacher or student, be sure that the new yogi is truly experiencing muscle soreness and not muscle pain. The two are quite different. If it is pain, then the student has gone "too far" and has entered overtraining mode.

4

Principle of Adaptation

According to this principle, the body adapts to the increased time or complexity of asanas in a highly specific way. By repeating the asana practice over and over again the body adapts, and the sequences or individual asanas become easier to perform. Wasn't it Pattabhi Jois who said, "Practice, practice, all is coming"? This principle explains why some beginning yogis are quite sore when starting a new yoga program – no matter the yoga style – but after doing it for a while, they feel there is much less muscle soreness associated with the program. As a yogini becomes comfortable with her yoga practice, she will need to vary the program to stay aligned with the principle of overload if she wants to continue to improve her strength, flexibility, balance, and stability.

5

Principle of Use/Disuse

This principle explains the idea of "use it or lose it." If you stop your physical asana practice, the gains in strength, flexibility, balance, ease, and elegance will also diminish. Listen to and follow your body to find out how much rest it needs.

6

Principle of Rest

When we rest, we give our bodies the opportunity to break from the "stress response" and take on the "relaxation response." To put it simply, we turn off the adrenaline output from the adrenal glands and allow for the body's physiology to return to normal.

By returning to normal, the digestive system works better at digestion, absorption, and elimination; the immune system works better at handling foreign and "sick" microbes; the muscular system relaxes and regenerates; and the system of fascia releases and unwinds. These are just a few examples of what happens physiologically with rest – a feeling much like getting topped up at the local gas station.

How often should I rest?

It all depends on your body, your health, and your practice. Some people need more rest to regenerate and recuperate than others. That is when it is time to return to listening to your body's signals – those spaced-out, spinny, frazzled, not-able-to-focus feelings while in asanas are a good sign that you have slipped into an adrenaline stressed-out state. It is time to move into a more restorative practice or to take a step away from the physical practice of yoga temporarily. When you return, your practice will feel as if you have had an oil change and are flowing with the best fuel in your system.

Summary

For each of us, these principles come from within the body, making up who we are. To follow them is a matter of listening closely to what the sensations of the body are saying. Be aware of whether your mind chatter or your body is running the show.

Principles of Movement Associated with Yoga Asanas

In addition to the foundational principles of physiology, there are eight foundational principles of movement that help prevent yoga injury while enabling you to delve deeper into your practice.

1. Nourish Relaxation

Relaxation

Relaxation is the state of mind that brings clarity and focus; it is the state in the body that generates muscle and fascia release, reduces pain, and generates strength. As it relates to yoga, it is the seed for cultivating dynamism. The more you can relax the safer, stronger, and more powerful your yoga practice will be.

Doing Nothing versus Effortless Effort

Relaxation has many different meanings that run the length of a spectrum. On one end is doing nothing. Doing nothing is what occurs when sitting on a beach chair sipping a drink with little umbrellas. At the other end is experiencing effortless effort. Effortless effort is conscious action while being at ease; it is strength cultivated from inner softness.

Cultivating Effortless Effort: Cultivating the Seeds of Relaxation for Dynamic Asanas

Effortless effort is initiated by being mindful – mindful of how the breath moves through the body and of the sensations that arise. Sensations can be anything including pain, tension, fatigue, strain, fullness, emptiness, ease, softness, and warmth. Once mindfulness is cultivated and the initial sensations and flow of breath felt, you can begin to relax into them, to feel breath and sensations as if you are immersed in them. As immersion continues, the sensations dissipate; a new layer of sensations emerges and the cycle begins again. As each new cycle of sensations emerges and dissipates there is a natural resolution, a natural rejuvenation. Within this resolution and rejuvenation lies dynamism.[1]

Elements of Relaxation: Soft, Easy Breathing Combined with Awareness Breathing

Relaxation that leads to effortless effort is initiated from within by soft and easy breathing. This type of breathing is nourishing, settling, calming, and quieting. It requires the mind to gently focus, to be aware of what is happening in the body. Being aware is to observe – just as you would observe a beautiful garden, landscape, or piece of art – taking it in without judgment. To experience this, try the following two-part exercise:

Part 1
Lie on your back and willfully breathe in deeply. Feel how your rib cage strongly expands and contracts as you inhale and exhale. How does this feel for you? Rest for a moment.

Part 2
We are now going to explore relaxation, which begins with imagination. Imagine your lungs sitting inside your rib cage. Two of them, each one filling either side of the rib cage, with the tops cresting the collarbones and the base of each nestling on top of the diaphragm (fig 3-1). As you breathe, feel the lung movement, the rising and falling. Notice how this rising and falling of the lungs causes the rib cage to rise and fall. Try not to use your will; let it occur from the inside out. As you let it occur from the inside out, you will probably feel your rib cage expanding more and with greater ease. You will also feel the exhalation becoming softer and calmer, as if you are on the top of a mountain allowing the breath to fill you – the lungs rise and fall softly, causing the rib cage to rise and fall softly. You will also notice less tension in your body. Now, if you would like, take this style of breathing into your practice and notice the degree of relaxation that emerges.

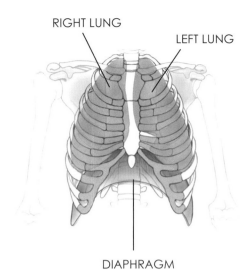

RIGHT LUNG

LEFT LUNG

DIAPHRAGM

Fig 3-1 Lungs and diaphragm

Physiology of Relaxation: The Nervous System

Although relaxation affects all aspects of the body's physiology, the primary system it works through is the nervous system. The nervous system can be considered the body's governing system since it activates the primary response to stressful or calming stimuli in the environment. If we perceive a stimulus to be stressful, the nervous system responds by inducing a sympathetic response called the fight, flight, or freeze response. When this type of response occurs, the body switches into high alert. When the nervous system perceives a calming response in the environment, it induces a parasympathetic response, or the relaxation response. In yoga, we want to induce this parasympathetic response. The optimal way to do this is to breathe softly, easily, and with awareness, then when we move, to connect our movement with the breath. One of the simplest ways to connect breath and movement is to begin with the spine in mind....

2. Initiate Movement: Begin with the Spine in Mind

The spine is the fundamental place to begin movement because of its central connection to every other piece of the body. Each of its vertebrae connects with fascia, blood vessels, muscles, and nerves, which in turn fan in various directions to nourish, stimulate, and balance each part of the body. At its essence, then, the spine is really a system of skeletal, neurological, electrical, vascular, and chemical input that when balanced and connected creates magically fluid movement, much the same way a well-balanced and connected orchestra creates awe-inspiring music.

This is important to keep in mind because we will be focusing mostly on the skeletal aspects of the spine as we delve deeper into the relationship between the spine and yoga asanas. As we do, allow the image of an orchestra to remain as a backdrop.[2]

Providing Balance: Stability and Mobility through Structure and Shape

Balance in Curves

Composed of 33 vertebrae arranged in four curves, the spine *(fig 3-2)* extends from the base of the skull to the bottom of the tailbone. From the skull to the tailbone, the curves are as follows:

- The cervical curve, consisting of 7 vertebrae.
- The thoracic curve, consisting of 12 vertebrae.
- The lumbar curve, consisting of 5 vertebrae.
- The sacral/coccygeal curve, consisting of 5 sacral vertebrae and 4 coccygeal vertebrae.

Of these four curves, only the cervical, thoracic, and lumbar curves contain movable vertebrae. The sacral vertebrae are fused together to form the sacrum, which as a unit can move on the 5th lumbar vertebra, which rests above, and the coccyx, which sits below. The coccygeal vertebrae are also fused. They create the coccyx, which as a unit can move on the sacrum above.

To describe the location of the vertebrae it is important to understand their abbreviations, which are a combination of a letter and a number. The letter refers to the curve that the similar shaped vertebrae reside in, and the number refers to the location within that curve. All of the vertebrae in the cervical curve start with "C"; the vertebrae in the thoracic curve start with "T"; the vertebrae in the lumbar curve start with "L"; and the vertebrae in the sacral curve start with "S." Therefore, since the cervical curve has 7 vertebrae, they are described as C1–C7. C5 would be the 5th vertebra from the top of the curve. The same occurs in the other curves:

- The 12 thoracic vertebrae are described at T1–T12.
- The 5 lumbar vertebrae are described at L1–L5.
- The 5 sacral vertebrae are described as S1–S5 (although since the sacrum consists of 5 fused vertebrae, in yoga we refer mostly to S1).

Together these four curves provide balance and fluidity of movement. They act as a coiled spring that imparts lightness by working as a shock absorber transferring and dissipating energy. If the curves didn't exist and if the spine were straight, it would move more like a tight, rigid wire – hard to move and unable to withstand the twisting, bending, and extension that we use in yoga asanas.

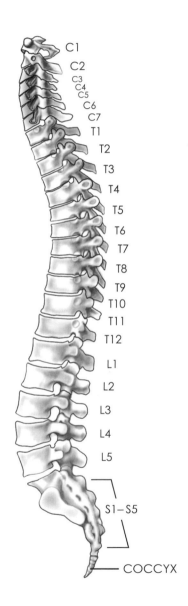

C1
C2
C3
C4
C5
C6
C7
T1
T2
T3
T4
T5
T6
T7
T8
T9
T10
T11
T12
L1
L2
L3
L4
L5
S1–S5
COCCYX

Fig 3-2 The spine

Stability in Stacking: The Spine as a Pyramid
(fig 3-3)

The spine is an incredibly grounded structure, impeccably designed to create a solid foundation. To get a feel for this, look at the spine from the back. Notice how in stacking the vertebrae bottom to top, the vertebrae become progressively smaller as your eye travels upward. Much like a pyramid, the spine has a wide base and a narrow top, giving the structure inherent stability.

Mobility within Each Segment: The Spine as a String of Pearls
(fig 3-3)

The spine is also exceptionally mobile. Its tiny vertebrae are joined as if they were pearls strung together to form a necklace, each pearl with its own independent movement.

Let's take this idea one step further. If each vertebral joint has its own independent movement, how much movement is truly available in the spine? An infinite amount!

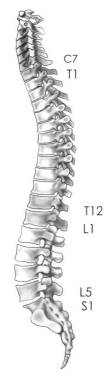

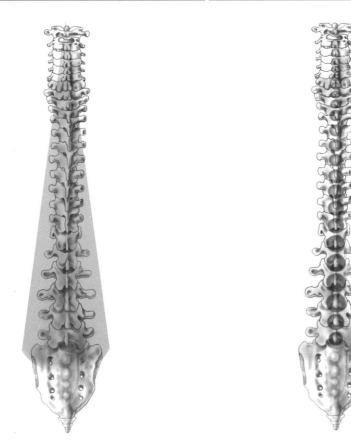

THE SPINE AS A PYRAMID

THE SPINE AS A STRING OF PEARLS

Fig 3-3 Visual analogies of the spine

Fig 3-4 The weak links of the spine at C7–T1, T12–L1, L5–S1

Then why do we have such problems at the spine if it is inherently stable and inherently mobile?

Part of the problem rests in whether we use our "will" to move or whether we use relaxation to move. When we move with our will, we increase tension in the body. When we increase tension in the body, movement becomes more difficult.

But there is more....

Weak Links: The Inherent Hypermobility of the Spine *(fig 3-4)*

Within the spine, each vertebral joint has its own range of movement. Some vertebral joints, however, allow more movement than others. These more movable joints are located at the junctions where the curves of the spine change direction:

- Between the cervical and thoracic curves at C7 and T1
- Between the thoracic and lumbar curves at T12 and L1
- Between the lumbar and sacral curves at L5 and S1

Our tendency as humans is to move in these areas more so than other areas. As a result these junctions become even more mobile while other parts of the spine become tighter, which leads to an increased risk for injury.[3]

How This Relates to Preventing Yoga Injuries

In yoga, students have a tendency to flare the lower ribs, jam through the lower back, or hinge at the lower neck. This is most noticeable in the lower back during back bends, in the neck during forward bends, and in the ribs when "bananaing" inversions and during twists. Students move this way because of habit, posture, and previous athletic endeavours. As a result, other vertebral joints become tighter or stuck – for example, between the scapulae in the thoracic curve or in the upper portion of the lumbar spine.

Ultimately then, in our yoga asanas, we want to improve movement of the vertebrae that tend to become stuck. As these vertebrae begin to move more easily, the more mobile areas of the spine no longer compensate for the tighter areas. Instead they take on a role of giving freedom, inviting ease, and re-creating space in the body.

This leads us to our next principle. Having maintained relaxation as we initiated movement from the spine, we can now go more deeply into an asana by connecting that spinal movement with movement at the largest joints first.

3. Connect Spinal Movement with Movement at the Largest Joints First

Once the body is relaxed and able to feel the spine as the place from which movement occurs, the next intention is to enable free and easy movement of the limbs. The simplest way to create this is by focusing on the largest joints first, specifically the shoulder and hip joints. This may be surprising to some yogis, since there are particular yoga systems that initiate movement at the hands and feet.

As they pertain to anatomical and kinesiological principles, the shoulder and hip joints are the most proximal, or the closest, to the spine, making it easier to maintain awareness and connect their movement to spinal movement.

The first step to creating connection between the spine and the shoulder joint, and the spine and the hip joint, is to understand the respective girdles that link them. These girdles are the shoulder girdle and the pelvic girdle.

The Shoulder Girdle

The shoulder girdle *(fig 3-5)* is a combination of bones, muscles, fascia, nerves, blood vessels, and joint capsules. As a group they work together to give the arms a large amount of support, mobility, and stability so that easy movement can occur – as when we raise and lower the arms in Surya Namaskar (Sun Salutation), or when we apply force and strength to the arms as in Chaturanga Dandasana (Four-Limbed Staff Pose) or Adho Mukha Svanasana (Downward Facing Dog).

 The softest things in the world overcome the hardest.

How the Shoulder Girdle Works: Joint Structure and Function

We'll begin our exploration of the bony aspects of the shoulder girdle from the front side. Have your hands free so that you can feel the pieces yourself. At the front are the clavicles. Each originates at the manubrium, the top portion of the sternum, at the sternoclavicular joint. Let your fingers linger here as you feel this "notch." From the sternum, move your fingers along as the clavicles expand wide toward the tip of each shoulder. You will feel the lateral end of the clavicles near the tip of each shoulder where they attach to the scapulae at the acromioclavicular joint. The *acromio* part of this joint refers to the acromion process of the scapula.

Go to the edge of the acromioclavicular joint and you will find the head of the humerus. The head of the humerus connects with the shoulder girdle at the glenoid fossa, which is the shallow cup of the scapula that faces laterally and slightly upward. The humerus connects into the glenoid fossa.

Moving to the back side from the glenoid fossa, you will feel the scapula resting on the back of the rib cage. Notice there is no bony joint attaching the scapula to the spine. Instead, attachment occurs through muscle onto the rib cage and onto the spine.

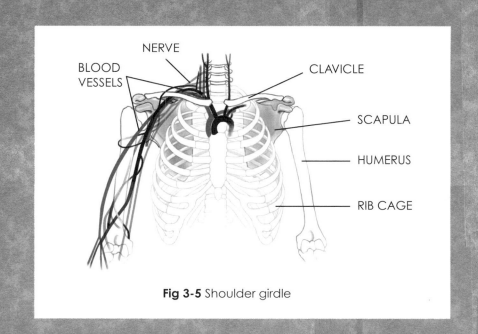

Fig 3-5 Shoulder girdle

Connecting the Spine, Shoulder Girdle, and Arm: Muscular Connection

The muscles that attach the shoulder girdle to the arm and the shoulder girdle to the spine can be considered collectively as the muscles that connect the arm to the torso. There are a lot of them. Some of these muscles provide stability, while others provide strength and power. Because of this, the exploration of the spine connecting to the shoulder girdle connecting to the arm is very interesting and intricate.

There are a few groups of muscles whose primary role is to stabilize the shoulder girdle to the spine and to stabilize the arm in the shoulder girdle so that movement is fluid, strong, and easy. For ease of learning, they have been divided into three groups. Shoulder stability is provided through the primary stabilizing structure, through the rotator cuff, and from the muscles and fascia in the deep front of the upper chest and shoulder.

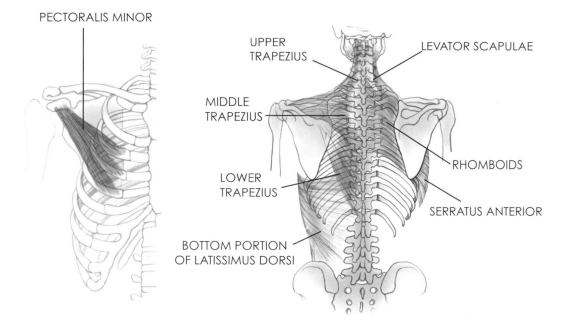

Fig 3-6 Primary stabilizing structure

The Primary Stabilizing Structure

The primary stabilizing structure *(fig 3-6)* consists of six muscles that connect the shoulder girdle to the rib cage and the spine. When these six muscles are balanced with each other, greater balance, stability, and flow of movement occur:

- The serratus anterior
- The major and minor rhomboids
- The lower, middle, and upper trapezius
- The levator scapulae
- The pectoralis minor
- The latissimus dorsi

Each of these muscles will be discussed in future sections of the book in different contexts. Just remember that to work effectively in each of their independent situations described later, they must be balanced with each other.

Together the balance of these muscles acts as an axis for movement, stability, strength, and mobility. The serratus anterior protracts the scapula so that it draws forward and underneath the armpit. It balances the rhomboids and middle trapezius, which retract the same scapula back toward the spine. The lower trapezius draws the scapula down the back toward the pelvis. It balances the upper trapezius and levator scapulae, which raise the scapula toward the ear as well as balance the pectoralis minor, which draws the scapula forward. Because the latissimus dorsi is a wide-spreading muscle originating from the thoracic and lumbar vertebrae, crossing over the inferior tip of the scapula, and attaching on the front side of the humerus, it helps connect the movement between the arm, scapula, spine, and pelvis by expanding the fluidity and balance of movement from the core stabilizing muscles outward. The latissimus dorsi depresses the shoulder girdle as well as moves the shoulder joint into extension, medial rotation, and adduction. Take a moment and feel these muscles on yourself or on someone else.

How each of these muscles interrelates will affect both the positioning of the scapula on the rib cage and the movement of the scapula as it relates to the arm. If one muscle is pulled tight or is weak, the scapula's ability to function optimally will be disrupted, leading to the possibility of injury in yoga asanas.

Stability through the Rotator Cuff

The rotator cuff *(fig 3-7)* is a group of four muscles that connect and stabilize the head of the humerus in the shoulder socket. They are well known to yoga instructors; many people come to yoga because of limited shoulder function as a result of a previous injury to the rotator cuff.

The four muscles that create the rotator cuff are the supraspinatus, infraspinatus, teres minor, and subscapularis. Together they control the shoulder at its socket as the arm moves through its large range of motion. The supraspinatus abducts the arm at the shoulder, the infraspinatus and teres minor externally rotate the arm at the shoulder, while the subscapularis adducts and medially rotates the arm at the shoulder.

But how does their action connect to the spine?

Four muscles physically link the rotator cuff to the spine via fascia – two of them connect to the cervical spine, and two of them connect to the thoracic spine.

Let's take a look:

Connecting to the cervical spine

The rotator cuff is linked, via fascia, to the cervical spine through the levator scapulae and the upper trapezius.[4] The levator scapulae and trapezius attach at the top of the scapula, and their fascia interweaves with the fascia of the supraspinatus. If either muscle is chronically tight or weak, the functioning of the rotator cuff will be affected, which in turn will affect the ability of the arm to move in all directions.

Connecting to the thoracic spine

The rotator cuff attaches to the thoracic spine through the rhomboids and latissimus dorsi.[5] The rhomboids attach to the medial border of the scapula, and the fascia links in with the fascia of the subscapularis. The latissimus dorsi attaches to the head of the front side of the humerus, with its fascia weaving together with the fascia of the infraspinatus and teres minor. The fascia is also connected at the ribs and inferior tip of the scapula. If either muscle is chronically tight or weak, the functioning of the rotator cuff will be affected, which in turn will affect the ability of the arm to move in all directions.

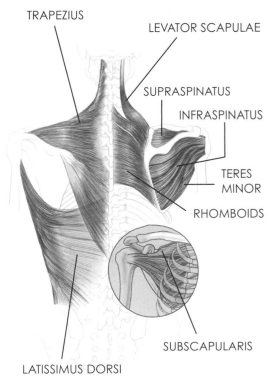

TRAPEZIUS

LEVATOR SCAPULAE

SUPRASPINATUS

INFRASPINATUS

TERES MINOR

RHOMBOIDS

SUBSCAPULARIS

LATISSIMUS DORSI

Fig 3-7 Connecting the action of the rotator cuff to the spine

Stability Deep in the Front of the Chest

A common posture that people hold is one of the shoulders rounded forward. When the shoulders are rounded forward, the functioning of the spine and the arm becomes affected.

Let's look deeper:

Going deep to the shoulder girdle, look at the scapula. You will notice that the scapula rests on the back of the rib cage. A little piece of bone sticks forward under the clavicle. That piece of bone, called the coracoid process, looks much like the beak of a crow, from which its name is derived. Three muscles attach to the coracoid process: the pectoralis minor, the biceps brachii, and the coracobrachialis. The pectoralis minor originates from the rib cage. The coraco-brachialis inserts onto the humerus, and the biceps brachii inserts onto the radius (fig 3-8).

Together they act as a group of linked chains, each affecting the other. If one muscle is tight, the other two will also be tight, and the head of the humerus will not be optimally centered in the glenoid fossa. As a result, the scapula elevates and pulls forward and the elbows bend. The influence doesn't end here. If these muscles are tight, causing the scapula to elevate, other muscles will try to respond to this, creating new tension, which in turn causes them to become tight as well. For example, it is a common pattern that when the pectoralis minor is tight, the levator scapulae is also tight (which can lead to dysfunction in both the cervical spine and rotator cuff, affecting the functioning of the arm). We will explore this further in inversions, which require a strong connection between the arm and the shoulder girdle.

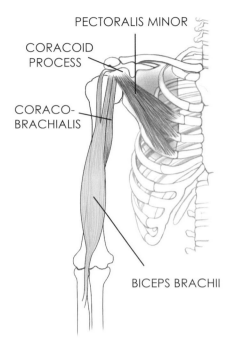

Fig 3-8 Stability deep in the front of the chest

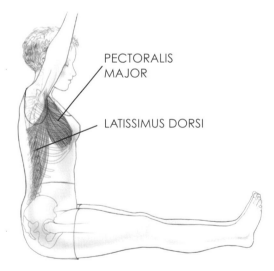

Fig 3-9 Strength and power from the front and side

Usually, Dandasana has the hands placed on the ground. The pressing of the hands into the ground activates the latissimus dorsi. This picture has the arms above so you can see the muscles.

Connecting the Spine, Shoulder Girdle, and Arm: Strength and Power

Once connection is clear between the spine and the muscles that create stability, power and strength can be developed. Strength and power are elicited from the muscles that are larger and more superficial.

Strength and Power from the Front and Side

Two key muscles work together to create strength and power: the pectoralis major and the latissimus dorsi (fig 3-9). We were introduced to the latissimus dorsi earlier as a primary stabilizing muscle because of how it connects the humerus to the scapula to the spine and pelvis. In this section, its role, in combination with the pectoralis major, is slightly different.

The pectoralis major is on the front of the body, originating on the sternum and the cartilage of the first six ribs as well as the medial half of the clavicle. It inserts on the crest of the greater tubercle of the humerus. As already explored, the latissimus dorsi covers a larger surface area, originating from the thoracic and lumbar vertebrae. Together these two muscles create a sling that connects the trunk and arm, enabling the trunk to lift upward as when climbing or when we sit in Dandasana (Staff Pose) in yoga.

Strength and Power from the Back and Side

The most superficial layer of muscle on the back is the trapezius muscle (fig 3-10). The trapezius covers a large area of the upper back, spanning from the base of the skull along each vertebra down to T12 and out to the acromion process and outer clavicle. Its fibers run in three different directions, enabling us to break the muscle into three sections – the upper trapezius, the middle trapezius, and the lower trapezius. Their importance is different depending on the asana and depending on the human who is creating the asana. As we explore the asanas specifically in the next section, we'll discuss this further.

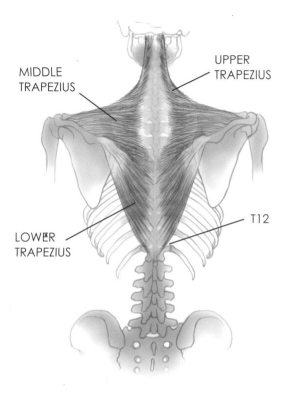

MIDDLE
TRAPEZIUS

UPPER
TRAPEZIUS

LOWER
TRAPEZIUS

T12

Fig 3-10 Trapezius muscle

How This Relates to Preventing Yoga Injuries

The action of muscles is much like a domino effect. If the vertebral joints in the cervical spine and/or the thoracic spine are tight, they will impede the functioning of the muscles that arise from them. In the previous examples, the muscles that arise from the cervical and/or thoracic spine are the levator scapulae, trapezius, rhomboids, pectoralis major, and latissimus dorsi. If these muscles are tight or weak, it will affect the body segment to which they connect. This chain reaction will occur all the way down to the wrist and hand. Therefore, tight and weak muscles of the shoulder girdle can affect the functioning of the hands and wrists.

How Weakness of the Shoulder Girdle and Upper Spine Can Affect Blood and Nerve Supply in the Wrist

While muscles can create "domino effects" from the upper spine and shoulder girdle down to the wrist and hand through their muscular connections, they can also create domino effects deeper in the body.

Directly under the pectoralis minor are nerves and blood vessels *(fig 3-11)*. When the muscles of the upper spine and shoulder girdle become tight or weak, causing the scapulae to rise up toward the ears and the shoulders to round forward, compression can occur in the front of the chest, just below the clavicles close to the armpits. Compression puts pressure on the nerves and blood vessels. When the nerves and blood vessels are under pressure, the flow of communication, nutrition, and oxygen is limited. Nerves tell the muscles how much and how fast to contract, and blood removes waste and rejuvenates the supply of oxygen. If either is limited in communication or delivery the muscles will fatigue faster. Carpal tunnel syndrome *(fig 3-12)* and other repetitive stress injuries then have greater potential to occur.

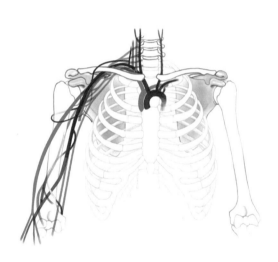

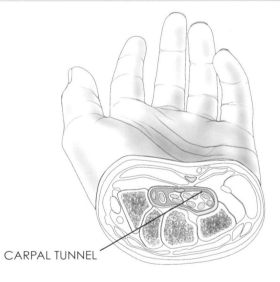

CARPAL TUNNEL

Fig 3-11 Arteries, veins, and skeletal components of the shoulder girdle

Fig 3-12 Carpal tunnel

When the muscles of the upper spine and shoulder girdle become tight or weak, causing the scapulae to rise up toward the ears and the shoulders to round forward, compression can occur in the front of the chest, just below the clavicles close to the armpits.

The Pelvic Girdle

The pelvic girdle is different in both structure and function from the shoulder girdle. The shoulder girdle provides a wide range of movement by acting as a support to hold the arms away from the body, whereas the pelvic girdle's design provides stability by keeping the legs close to and underneath the body. As a result, the primary purpose of the pelvic girdle is to carry and transfer weight from the spine to the legs for walking, standing, running, and climbing.

How the Pelvic Girdle Works: Joint Structure and Function

The pelvic girdle consists of two large pelvic bones attached to the sacrum in the back and the pubic symphysis in the front *(fig 3-13)*. On the lateral side of each pelvic bone is the acetabulum. The acetabulum connects with the femur to create the hip joint.

Let's take a further look at the pelvic bone. The pelvic bone has a very distinct shape. It is somewhat round, somewhat flat, and definitely irregular in shape. Upon closer examination, your eye will probably notice that it is not just one bone; it is three bones fused together. These three bones are the ilium, the pubis, and the ischium.

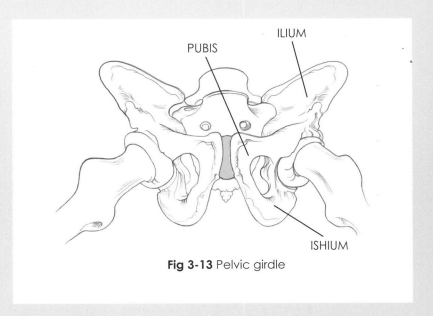

Fig 3-13 Pelvic girdle

The ilium

Begin in a seated position with your hands on your hips. You will feel the top of your two hip bones as a ridge under your fingers. This is the iliac crest. As you move forward along the crest, it will feel as if you were walking along the ridge of a mountain, with your fingers sliding side to side. As you move along the ridge, you will reach a distinctive edge. It will feel like a "sticky outy." This "sticky outy" protrudes forward and is called the anterior superior iliac spine (ASIS). Let your fingers slip medially over the edge and plunge into the muscles and tissue that rest in the bowl of your pelvis. Take your thumbs and rest them on the lateral side of the ASIS. You are holding onto the hip bone. This is the ilium.

If you follow your hands around to the back of the ilium toward the sacrum, you will come in contact with the sacroiliac (SI) joint. This is the joint that joins the ilium to the sacrum.

The pubis

Now place one hand on your lower belly, with the heel of your hand at your navel and your fingers pointing downward. Press gently and deeply with your middle finger. You will be either on or very near the pubic symphysis. This is the joint that connects the body of the pubis of each pelvic bone. If you palpate firmly and deeply, you will feel how from the pubic symphysis, the pubis moves posteriorly, laterally, and inferiorly to join with the ilium and ischium to form the acetabulum.

The ischium

The ischium is the base of the pelvis. When sitting, place your hands under your bum and rest all of your weight in your hands. The bone you feel in each of your hands is your ischium. Keep palpating through your bum muscles to feel how the ischium creates the lower part of the pelvis. In many practices, yogis move their butt cheeks to sit directly on the ischial tuberosities of the ischium, hence the name *sitting bones*, the common term used to describe this area.

Connecting the Spine, Pelvic Girdle, and Leg: Stability, Mobility, and Strength

Since the purpose of the pelvic girdle is to transfer weight and energy from the spine to the legs its role is like that of a bridge. The role of the muscles, then, is to help maintain the stability of the bridge function while also affording the femur mobility, stability, strength, and power.

Stability from Several Directions: Posteriorly, Medially, and Laterally

Stability of the pelvis comes from several directions. One is from the back side in the form of the external rotators, another is from the inside in the form of the hip adductors, and the other is from the outside in the form of the hip abductors. Together these muscles work as a functional synergy to bridge the connection from the spine, through the pelvis, and onto the femur.

Hip external rotators (also known as lateral rotators)

There are six external rotators (fig 3-14) that attach on the pelvis and on the femur. Depending on the text and the author, there is some discussion and disagreement on whether all six of these muscles are true external rotators, as well as which of the six are considered to be the primary movers. Here are the fundamentals.

The piriformis is perhaps the best known of the lateral rotators because of its size (it is the largest of the six) and its proximity to the sciatic nerve. The piriformis is the only external rotator that attaches to the spine at the sacrum. It lines the back and lateral sides of the pelvis, creating a "posterior and lateral pelvic wall.[6] The obturator internus and the gemellus superior and inferior gather and blend together on the inside of the pelvis and attach onto the femur. The obturator externus and quadratus femoris are sometimes considered external rotators and sometimes not; however, since both help stabilize the connection between the pelvis and the femur, we'll keep them in the group of external rotators for this exploration.

Collectively, for the sake of understanding their action in yoga asanas, the external rotators all help maintain the connection of the spine, pelvis, and leg. Some of them are known to externally rotate the leg bone, and all of them stabilize the pelvis on the femur by keeping the femur head in the acetabulum.

Hip abductors

From the outside, the hip abductors (fig 3-15) create a connection of support by steadying the pelvis when we are standing on one or two legs. Collectively, these muscles prevent the front knee from falling inward when in standing poses. They are the gluteus medius, the gluteus minimus, and the tensor fascia latae, which leads into the iliotibial band. The piriformis and obturator externus also act as secondary abductors to steady the pelvis.

Hip adductors

The hip adductors (fig 3-16) are a group of five muscles that make up the musculature of the inner thigh. They are the pectineus, the adductor magnus, the gracilis, the adductor brevis, and the adductor longus. In connecting the inner thigh bone to the pelvis, their primary role is to bring the legs together.

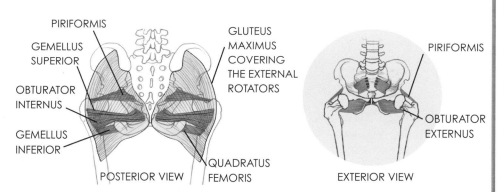

PIRIFORMIS
GEMELLUS SUPERIOR
OBTURATOR INTERNUS
GEMELLUS INFERIOR
GLUTEUS MAXIMUS COVERING THE EXTERNAL ROTATORS
QUADRATUS FEMORIS
POSTERIOR VIEW
PIRIFORMIS
OBTURATOR EXTERNUS
EXTERIOR VIEW

Fig 3-14 Hip external rotators

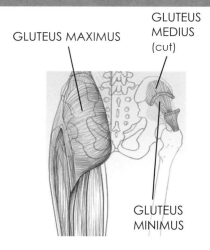

GLUTEUS MAXIMUS
GLUTEUS MEDIUS (cut)
GLUTEUS MINIMUS

Fig 3-15 Hip abductors

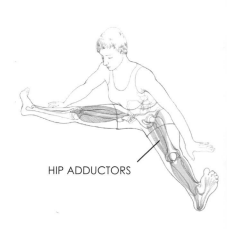

HIP ADDUCTORS

Fig 3-16 Hip adductors

Strength and Power

Once the connection between the hip external rotators, hip abductors, and hip adductors is working functionally, power and strength can develop. The chief power muscle connecting the pelvis to the spine is the gluteus maximus. It is the largest and most superficial muscle in the buttocks. Two of its primary roles are to externally rotate and extend the femur. A third role that isn't spoken about as much arises through its attachment to the iliotibial band. Remember that the tensor fascia latae also attaches to the iliotibial band. Together the gluteus maximus and the tensor fascia latae bring balance to the iliotibial band, which contributes to stability of the knee (fig 3-17) – an important component when balancing on one leg such as in Vrksasana (Tree Pose).

This leads us to our next principle. Now that we have connected the spine and the movement of the largest joints first, we need to be sure to move the joints optimally. If we move too far injury can occur; if we do not move far enough, then the full benefit of the yoga practice is not enjoyed. Read on to explore how to distinguish if you are moving your joints in their optimum range of motion.

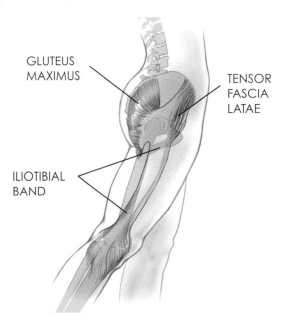

GLUTEUS
MAXIMUS

TENSOR
FASCIA
LATAE

ILIOTIBIAL
BAND

Fig 3-17 Strength and power of the hips

4. Move Joints in Their Optimum Range of Motion

All joints have their own optimum range of motion. Some move more, such as the shoulder and hip joints; others move less, such as the sacroiliac joint. Even between bodies there is an optimum range of motion. One person may have arthritic or swollen joints, while another may have very healthy joints that have never been injured. Different situations create different ranges of motion, so to ensure injury doesn't occur, the key is to move only as far as the joint allows – whether arthritic or healthy. If movement is forced beyond that point, tearing, straining, pulling, or breaking is possible, and other joints may have to compensate.

How do I know if my joints are moving in their optimum range of motion?

- You are relaxed.
- You can breathe.
- The joint is moving in a direction it is designed to move in.
- You feel no pain (see principle 7).

Now that the joints are moving, the next principle can be introduced. Core stability is foundational for bringing lightness and ease into yoga asanas. Read on for more….

5. Develop Core Stability: Boost Up Your Bandhas and Breathe

Some people move through yoga asanas with a grace and ease that is fluid, gently strong, and very relaxed. It is as if their strength of calmness permeates from the core of their bodies to the tips of their fingers, to the tips of their toes, and softly out of their bodies.

This is the essence of core stability.

The body is like a boat on water, where the body is the boat and the external stimulus is the water. Both are stable and able to respond to the inevitable wobbles, turns, and shifts only when they are balanced. In the body, this balance enables us to move from slow to fast and fast to slow; it gives a strength and ease to movement whether or not the limbs are involved; it lets us know where our bodies are in space; it ensures our foundations are stable while our body parts move in a coordinated flow.[7]

Core stability is a balance of strength and mobility – the balance of strong core muscles, found along the midline of the body from the base of the skull to the bottom of the feet, combined with freedom of movement of the hip, shoulder, and vertebral joints as well as the elbow, knee, wrist, and ankle joints. Without this balance, the body will either be too rigid (too much strength with too little mobility) or limp and spiritless (too much mobility with too little strength).

The body is like a boat on water, where the body is the boat and the external stimulus is the water. Both are stable and able to respond to the inevitable wobbles, turns, and shifts only when they are balanced.

Creating Core Stability in Yoga Asanas

The beauty of yoga as it relates to core stability is that core stability has been inherently part of the practice.

As explored previously, core stability is a combination of strength and mobility. The strength component requires muscle balance along the midline of the body, from the base of the skull to the bottom of the feet. In yoga, this can be created through the bandhas.

The bandhas are energetic locks located at specific locations in the body. Although they are energetic, they can be accessed through our physical anatomy. In this book we'll explore five bandhas:

Three primary bandhas

- Mula bandha in the pelvis
- Uddiyana bandha just beneath the navel
- Jalandara bandha in the area of the neck

Two secondary bandhas

- Pada bandha in the feet
- Hasta bandha in the hands

The three primary bandhas (fig 3-18) will be explored in this section, while the secondary bandhas, pada bandha and hasta bandha, will be explored in standing poses and inversions, respectively.

1

Mula Bandha

Mula bandha is situated in the pelvis. Its location is slightly different in men and women. For men, it is the area between the scrotum and the anus, two inches inside the body. For women, it is located by the cervix.

Let's find it:

Sit or lie down. Completely relax and bring your awareness to the pelvis. If you are a woman, bring your attention to the opening of the vagina. Move up the vagina toward the cervix, which is the opening of the uterus. Breathing easily, allow your attention to gently focus. Contract the muscles so that you feel this area a little more. Be gentle. Remember the feeling.

If you are a man, bring your attention to between your anus and scrotum. Gently lift your scrotum into your body, without bearing down. Gently focus on where you feel the lift, breathing easily. Remember the feeling.[8]

Now that you've pinpointed the feeling of mula bandha, let's explore the anatomy related to it. We'll begin at the pelvic floor and move downward.

The Pelvic Floor

The pelvic floor is an intricate array of muscles, fascia, blood vessels, and nerves. The muscles and fascia are arranged in layers and in different directions. We'll be exploring two layers – the perineum and the pelvic diaphragm.

JALANDARA BANDHA

TRANSVERSUS ABDOMINIS

area of:
UDDIYANA BANDHA

MULA BANDHA

HIP ADDUCTORS

TIBIALIS POSTERIOR
(shaded in behind)

PERONEUS LONGUS

Fig 3-18 The primary bandhas and their associated muscles

The perineum

The perineum as an anatomical term is different from the yogic term. In yoga, the perineum is the area between the genitals and anus. In anatomy, the perineum includes the space between the genitals and anus plus more. Shaped like a diamond, it has the pubic symphysis at the front, the coccyx at the back, and the ischial tuberosities left and right.

The perineum is further divided into an anterior and posterior triangle. The anterior triangle is known as the urogenital triangle, and the posterior triangle is known as the anal triangle. Having knowledge of the anatomical definition will give greater understanding of the muscles involved.

Within the urogenital triangle is the urogenital diaphragm, which is created by deep and superficial muscles. The deep muscles are the transverse perineal muscles. The superficial muscles are the superficial transverse perineal muscles, which connect the two ischial tuberosities; the bulbospongiosus, which surrounds the vagina in women and the bulb of the penis in men; and the ischiocavernosus, which connects the ischium to the clitoris in women and covers the penile crura in men.

The pelvic diaphragm

The pelvic diaphragm is shaped much like a funnel or hammock. Separating the pelvic cavity from the perineum, it is composed primarily of the levator ani and the coccygeus muscles. It covers or closes most of the opening of the pelvis except for the area around the prostate in men and the vagina in women, where the fascia of the urogenital diaphragm resides.

When creating mula bandha from the muscles of the pelvis, three primary muscles are contracting. These are the muscles of the urogenital diaphragm:

- Superficial and deep transverse perineal muscles
- Bulbospongiosus muscle
- Ischiocavernosus muscle

Accessing Mula Bandha from Below

The initiatory action of mula bandha is not isolated to the pelvic floor. Let's explore further:

Hip adductors

The hip adductor muscles *(fig 3-18)* have a fascial connection to the pelvic floor muscles and through their gentle contraction can stimulate the transverse perineal and bulbospongiosus muscles to contract.

Fibularis (peroneus) longus and tibialis posterior

Attaching to the fibula, the fibularis (peroneus) longus is located on the lateral side of the leg. It moves down the fibula, around the lateral malleolus, and attaches on the bottom of the foot. The tibialis posterior attaches to the posterior side of the tibia and fibula as well as to the membrane between the tibia and fibula. It angles medially, wraps around the medial malleolus, and attaches on the bottom of the foot. Together, the fibularis (peroneus) longus and tibialis posterior act as a stirrup. With sprawling attachments on the bottom of the feet they lift the arches. Their fascial attachments on the fibula and tibia connect with the fascial attachments of the hip adductors. It is this connection that enables the feet to contribute to creating mula bandha and core stability *(fig 3-18)*.

2

Uddiyana Bandha
Uddiyana bandha is located about three inches below the navel in both men and women.

Let's find it:

While lying on your back, bring your attention to three inches below your navel. Gently draw this area in toward your core. Be sure you are not contracting above your navel, and don't hold your breath. Move only the spot three inches below your navel.[9]

Now that you've pinpointed the feeling of uddiyana bandha, let's explore the anatomy related to it.

Uddiyana bandha feeds off of mula bandha *(fig 3-18)*. It is the activation of mula bandha along with the contraction of the transversus abdominis, the lower fibers of the internal oblique, and multifidi muscles *(fig 3-18)*.

The transversus abdominis is the innermost muscle of the abdomen, covering the area from the rib cage to the pelvis. At the rib cage it attaches to the lower ribs and interweaves with the diaphragm. In the pelvis it attaches to the pubis. Its fibers run horizontally, so it also attaches around the back to the lumbodorsal fascia as well as in the front to the linea alba. When the fibers contract they act like a girdle, squeezing into the core of the body.

The internal oblique works in conjunction with the transversus abdominis. While the fibers of the internal oblique span from the pelvis to the rib cage, only the lower fibers work in conjunction with the transversus abdominis. The lower fibers attach to the iliac crest of the pelvis near the anterior superior iliac spine. They also attach with the transversus abdominis onto the pubis and onto the linea alba. When they contract, they contract with the transversus abdominis, supporting and compressing into the core of the body.

The muscles of mula bandha and the transversus abdominis work closely with the multifidi. The multifidi are small muscles that attach between vertebrae, spanning the entire spine from the sacrum to C2. Specifically, they attach from the transverse process of one vertebra to the spinous process three or four vertebrae higher.

Mula Bandha, Uddiyana Bandha, Core Stability, and the Anal Muscles

Learning core stability from the pelvic floor muscles can be challenging, no matter if it is explored through mula bandha or other means. Sometimes, to make learning easier, the concept is taught by contracting the anal muscles first. This may give beginners greater confidence in finding what they are supposed to be contracting, but it can be dangerous. A direct connection exists between mula bandha and uddiyana bandha. The two flow together, both energetically and anatomically. When the anal muscles are contracted, the muscular contractions joining the two bandhas are destroyed, and core stability is lost. This is due to the neural connection between the muscles connecting the core. It is best to practice both mula bandha and uddiyana bandha without contracting the anal muscles.

3

Jalandara Bandha
Jalandara bandha is located in the neck.

Let's find it:

Take a rolled up elastic bandage, a small orange, or a tennis ball and hold onto it with just your neck. Don't clench, and allow only your head to move forward on your spine. This feeling is jalandara bandha.[10] Let's explore further:

The muscles of jalandara bandha are commonly called the deep neck flexors, also known as the longus colli, longus capitis, rectus capitis anterior, and rectus capitis lateralis. The longus colli and longus capitis are more medial to the spine than the rectus capitis anterior and rectus capitis lateralis.

The longus colli attaches from the anterior side of C1 down to T3. The longus capitis attaches from the transverse processes of the cervical vertebrae to the base of the skull.

The rectus capitis anterior is wider and shorter than the longus colli and capitis. It attaches from C1 to the base of the skull. As the name implies, the rectus capitis lateralis is more lateral to the spine than the rectus capitis anterior. It attaches from the transverse process of C1 to the skull.

Together these four muscles help balance the head on the spine and gently drop the chin into jalandara bandha.

How This Relates to Preventing Yoga Injuries

In yoga, core stability enables us to flow from asana to asana without getting injured. It enables us to hold an asana statically then suddenly jump our feet between our hands. It allows us to radically shift our body position from a back bend to a forward bend/inversion, as when moving from Urdhva Mukha Svanasana (Upward Facing Dog) into Adho Mukha Svanasana (Downward Facing Dog). It gives us the ease and strength needed to stay in an asana for an extended period of time.

The Relationship of the Bandhas to Breathing

Yoga, as a system of exercises, is designed to balance and create space within the body. Within that space, energy is transformed into prana, our life force. Core stability, or the activation of the bandhas, is an important component in creating and maintaining that space. However, since we are activating the bandhas via our physical anatomy, there can be a tendency to overcontract, bear down, or push too hard in the activation. As a result, more tension is created and less stability and strength is experienced. Grace and ease, poise and elegance become less tangible as feelings. Instead, pain, injury, and dysfunction become possible, albeit unwanted, alternatives.

So what to do?

Stability and strength are generated from relaxation. Relaxation is initiated by breathing easily, calmly, and fluidly. So, in order to nurture and develop core stability, it is necessary to breathe easily, calmly, and fluidly throughout yoga asanas.

Let's experience this:

Experience for a moment the feelings of holding your breath. Move into any yoga asanas while holding your breath. Keep your breath held as you move in and out of the asanas. Notice what you feel. Then, move in and out of the asanas with a calm, easy, and fluidly moving breath. Do you feel the pose differently – lighter perhaps?

How does this work?

Breathing is the element that connects all of our movements. The bones, muscles, and connective tissue may create structure, but breath is the ebb and flow of that structure. When it is fluid, it brings life. When it is held, it can stiffen or even collapse our movements.

Breathing smoothes out our lines. It takes the balance of strength and mobility necessary for core stability and augments it by infusing poise and grace. Without breathing, core stability is really just constipated rigidity.

Elements of Breath

Breathing occurs as the result of many components of the respiratory system working together – mouth, nose, trachea, bronchi, lungs, bronchioles, alveoli, and diaphragm.

Let's experience how they work together:

Lie on your back.

Feel yourself breathing. Feel the air entering your nose. Feel your lungs expanding into your rib cage. Feel the respiratory diaphragm dropping and lifting. Feel your abdomen rising and falling in concert with the diaphragm rising and falling.

Let's move more subtly.

As you feel your breath, feel into your pelvis. Feel the gentle movement of your pelvic floor dropping as you inhale and lifting as you exhale. Feel how the sensation of the movement can be felt down into your toes.

How does this relate to the rest of the body?

We'll look at the impact of breathing on core stability through the diaphragm (fig 3-19). The diaphragm is often considered the primary breathing muscle. Located in the rib cage, its position divides the body almost in half. The heart and lungs rest above, while the pancreas, stomach, gallbladder, spleen, liver, intestines, and reproductive organs lie below. To connect these organs above and below there are orifices, or holes, in the diaphragm to allow for vessels to pass through.

The diaphragm can be divided into two parts. One part is dome shaped and resides just behind the xiphoid process of the sternum and the lower six ribs. The second part, called the crura, looks like a handle. It attaches to the first two or three lumbar vertebrae.

Whenever I feel blue,
   I start breathing again.

— *L. Frank Baum*

The movement of the diaphragm has a direct impact on core stability for two reasons:

1

When the diaphragm is moving well, most of the time breath is moving well. This enables the relaxation response to occur in the body. Core stability is greatly enhanced when this response, rather than the adrenalized stress response, is turned on.

2

The second reason is the connection of the diaphragm to the surrounding muscles and fascia.

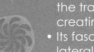

- The attachment point of the diaphragm at the bottom six ribs is also the attachment point for the transversus abdominis, the key muscle for creating core stability.
- Its fascial connection to the ribs around the lateral and posterior sides of the rib cage connects with the fascia of the serratus anterior.
- The diaphragm's crura have an attachment point at the first two or three lumbar vertebrae. This is the same attachment point as the psoas.

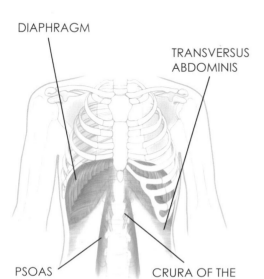

DIAPHRAGM

TRANSVERSUS ABDOMINIS

PSOAS

CRURA OF THE DIAPHRAGM

Fig 3-19 The diaphragm, its crura and the psoas

When the breath is held, it will have a direct negative impact on the movement and functioning of the transversus abdominis, which will impede the full experience of core stability, which limits access to the bandhas, which creates rigid yoga asanas that develop external strength and tension at the expense of internal stability, relaxation, and ease.

Although we didn't explore the psoas or serratus anterior as they relate to core stability, when the breath is held they may also be held, which will affect the dynamic state of equilibrium in the body.

Now that you've renewed and rejuvenated through mobility, stability, and breath, it is time to go deeper into asanas – to take the ideas learned intellectually and feel them viscerally; to experience strength as relaxation and to experience relaxation as resiliency. Read on to learn how in the next principle.

 Learn to be calm and you'll always be happy.

6. Adopt Relaxed Resilience

Relaxation occurs in a cycle of layers. It begins with breath and continues with awareness. For example, many people start a yoga practice with breathing in either a sitting, standing, or reclining position. As the breathing rate, depth, and ease are observed, the beginning stages of relaxation are induced, and the parasympathetic nervous system response is turned on. Awareness develops. As awareness develops, a yogi can perceive the level of tension or freedom that exists in his muscles, connective tissue, or joints. If tension is perceived, the yogi can use his breath to release it.

As the practice continues, movement occurs – either in the form of a sequenced vinyasa practice or in the form of statically held asanas. Whichever the form, the cycle continues – observation of breath, which results in relaxation, which leads to body awareness.

Breathing, relaxing, and developing awareness enable you to feel and connect to your anatomy and physiology. It takes the learning of anatomy from the cerebral level to the body level, from knowing it intellectually to understanding it viscerally. It brings balance and helps mobilize joints. It facilitates circulation and improves strength, coordination, and communication between the nerves and muscles. It makes you sensitive so that you can feel what is blocked in your body and then be able to do something about it rather than force through it, which could potentially cause injury. Not being relaxed and aware is a recipe for trouble.

Relaxation in yoga asanas is not "doing nothing." It is the direct experience of the vital and dynamic action that is inside, which occurs when there is space and freedom for movement. It occurs when we don't force the movement. When movements in yoga asanas are forced, tension develops. Typically, the tension develops at the superficial layers of muscles. As relaxation develops, the superficial muscles can release, and deeper muscles can take over. As a result, core stability improves, mobility and flexibility increase, and strength and power are enhanced. That is relaxed resilience.

Relaxed resilience can only be experienced with easy, fluid breathing and awareness, when the first principle of movement – relaxation – is applied to the second, third, fourth, and fifth principles of movement – begin with the spine in mind, connect spinal movement with movement at the largest joints first, move joints in their optimum range of motion, and develop core stability. As a result, the asanas, whether held statically or sequenced in a vinyasa flow, become a practice that feels like effortless effort. Relaxed resilience is effortless effort.

Let's consider a common example:

As students start out in yoga, their first awareness may be that their scapulae sit by their ears. They might not have realized that before, but after a few classes their awareness of this fact develops. As they continue to practice, they feel a release and begin to experience freedom and a new strength around their spine, shoulders, and scapulae. They begin to experience a new pattern of movement – not one that they forced on themselves but rather one that emerged naturally.

This leads us to the next principle. Sometimes the "will" can get the best of us and take us too far, too fast. The next principle helps you be generous and move in your pain-free range of motion.

7. Be Generous with Yourself: Move in Your Pain-Free Range of Motion

Pain. This is a loaded word with many meanings and interpretations. What pain is and how it is felt depend on the person experiencing it; what one person finds painful and what another person finds painful could be described and felt in very different ways. So, for the sake of clarity, let's describe pain along a spectrum. Good pain on one side, bad pain on the other, with a host of nondescriptive aches, twinges, and feelings in between.

"Good pain" is the discomfort caused by muscle fatigue. Muscle fatigue is the point at which the muscle fibers can no longer contract. Nerves are still stimulating the fibers to contract, but the fibers aren't responding – either because they have exhausted their energy reserves or there is a buildup of lactic acid.[11] This is good. Strength can be developed as a result of muscle fatigue, or "good pain."

On the other end of the spectrum is bad pain – the pain that sears, tears, strains, and rips; the pain that makes people wonder why they signed up. It is the pain that continues to be sensitive five or six days after a yoga class. It is also the pain that causes your forehead or brow to furrow, your jaw to clench, and your breath to become shallow, held, and tense. This type of pain is not beneficial for developing body balance. Rather, this kind of pain increases tension in the body, causing fluid, easy breath to become constrained and constricted, muscle and fascia to contract forcefully, and tension to reverberate through the body. When experiencing pain in this way, mobility and strength will decrease.

Delayed Onset Muscle Soreness

Delayed onset muscle soreness (DOMS) is the experience of feeling muscle soreness two or even three days after your yoga session. You may be surprised to feel sore, especially if you didn't feel muscle discomfort or muscle fatigue while you were moving through the yoga asanas. If you are experiencing DOMS, it usually goes away by the fourth day following the yoga session. An easy yoga practice with a focus on breathing and relaxation will help excrete the lactic acid and other physiological waste products that cause this type of soreness.

Now, we can move into the final principle – less is always more. Have fun reading!

8. Less Is More: Develop Strength, Stability, Mobility, and Flexibility in the Simple Yoga Asanas Before Moving into the Complex Yoga Asanas

Less is more is not an unfamiliar concept. Start small, take baby steps, and bite off no more than you can chew all describe the same concept in a different way. When learning new yoga asanas, whether as a beginning yogini or an experienced yogini, you will always gain more when you take on smaller amounts in the form of simple yoga asanas before moving into complex yoga asanas.

Simple yoga asanas are different from complex yoga asanas because they use fewer joint movements. For example, Dandasana (Staff Pose) is a simple yoga asana. Both legs are doing the same thing at their respective hip joints. Balance is straightforward to create. To make this more complex, we can move into Marichyasana (Pose Dedicated to the Sage Marichi). From Dandasana a twist has been added, along with a different position between the left and right sides. The arms are also being used to help leverage the spine into a rotation. In the twist there is potential for the pelvis to move out of balance, which means the potential for strain and injury is also greater.

Since the potential for moving out of balance – or moving into strain – is greater in complex yoga asanas, it is important to have gained the mobility, stability, strength, and flexibility in the simple asanas before moving on in order to prevent yoga injuries.

Now that the principles of movement have been explored, let's get into the meat of yoga asanas.

 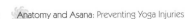

wind

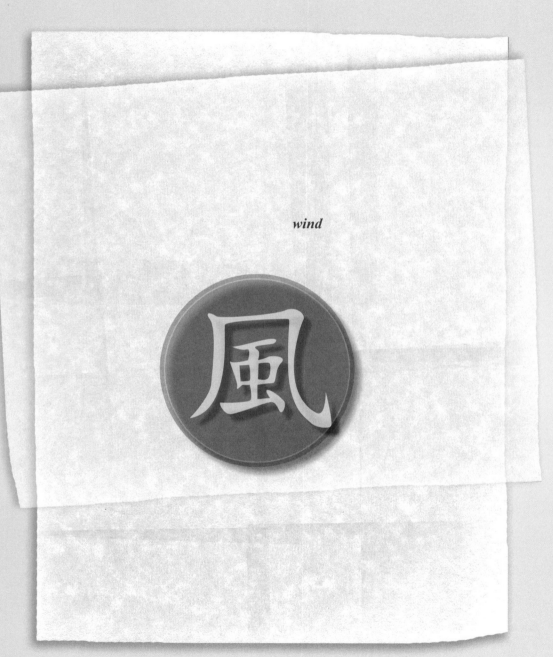

Breathe. Let go. And remind yourself

that this very moment is the only one

you know you have for sure.

— *Oprah Winfrey*

asana

Standing poses are grounding.

Standing poses are powerfully grounding. With one or two feet on the ground, they can move the body in all sorts of directions. As a group of poses, they tie together the delicious qualities of back bends, the graciousness that enfolds forward bends, the delight of twists, and the lightness that imbues inversions. Standing poses are powerful, yet they subtly connect the parts of the body from the spine outward – from the spine into the pelvis, legs, and feet; and from the spine into the shoulder girdle and out to the arms and hands. In doing so, not only do they train us for all the other yoga asanas, they also train us for our most basic day-to-day activities including standing still, walking, bending forward, sitting down, and standing back up again.

As a beginning yoga student, I remember my teacher telling me that Tadasana was the foundational position of all yoga asanas. I have to admit, I thought she was crazy. Then we moved into Vrksasana (Tree Pose) and into Garudasana (Eagle Pose), then into Virabhadrasana 3 (Warrior 3 Pose). Since I was able to do each of these poses, her Tadasana teachings meant nothing to me. But I knew something was missing. My teacher would come by and tell me to "feel the rhythm of your Tadasana feet, and a sense of softness and ease will balance your hardness." Still, for a long time I had no idea what she was talking about. Then just a few years ago, I got it. I began to understand the dynamic interplay between firmness and suppleness, which together create the rhythm of the feet, the lightness in the standing pose, and the ease in the inversion.

Standing poses are superb for developing strength in the legs, mobility in the hips, and coordination between the spine and the shoulder and pelvic girdles. In doing so, they connect the major pieces of the body. However, if the pieces are out of balance with each other, then problems can occur. Segmental instability between the lumbar spine and pelvis can lead to pain and irritation in the knees; poor core stability can create problems in the hips and in the shoulders; spinal tightness as it relates to the rib cage or scapulae can affect the movement of the arms. So it is important to begin by relaxing first and *then* moving – and when you do initiate movement, begin with the spine in mind.

Standing Poses, the Spine, and the Feet

Standing poses bring lightness to the spine by way of strength in the legs, and strength in the legs can be influenced by the feet. How the feet are positioned and their relative flexibility and resiliency will impact the action of the legs, which will influence how the spine responds and moves. Likewise, how the spine is functioning will also have an impact on the functioning of the legs and the positioning, flexibility, and resiliency of the feet.

Let's take a look:

The positioning of the spine in standing poses is not consistent. Depending on the asana, the spine can be neutral, perpendicular to the floor or neutral yet parallel to the floor. It can also be in flexion, extension, or rotation. How smoothly the spine moves into its various positions depends on how the feet stabilize and balance.

It is important to note the obvious here – there are a few bones between the spine and the feet that also need to be considered: the pelvic bones, femurs, tibias, and fibulas. So in considering the key movements of the feet and spine in standing poses, we also need to consider the movements of the hip sockets, knees, and ankles.

The Variety of Standing Poses: The Permutations and Combinations of the Spine, Legs, and Arms

When looking at the positioning of the limbs, there are several different variations of standing poses.

The legs have five:

- Legs and feet together, as in Tadasana (Mountain Pose)
- Feet apart, both feet pointing in the same direction, as in Prasarita Padottanasana (Wide-Legged Forward Bend)
- Feet apart, pointing in two different directions, with the front knee bent, as in Virabhadrasana 1 and 2 (Warrior 1 and 2 Pose)
- Feet apart, pointing in two different directions, with both legs straight, as in Trikonasana (Triangle Pose)
- Only one foot on the ground, as in Vrksasana (Tree Pose)

Arm position also varies in poses:

- Overhead, as in Virabhadrasana 1 (Warrior 1 Pose)
- In abduction, as in Virabhadrasana 2 (Warrior 2 Pose)
- In front, as in Garudasana (Eagle Pose)
- Behind, as in Parsvottanasana (Pyramid Pose)

Combine the various arm and leg positions, along with the variety of spinal movements, and several permutations and combinations of the body are possible in standing poses. Even so, there are commonalities to each of the positions. We will break them down by looking first at the lower body and then at the upper body.

How the Lower Body Works in Standing Poses

Since the foundational position in yoga asanas is Tadasana (Mountain Pose) *(fig 4-1)*, we'll begin our exploration here. Tadasana requires us to stand on our feet, with toes facing forward. To do this softly, strongly, and with ease requires a few key elements:

- The heads of the femurs settle into the acetabulum of the pelvis.
- The condyles of the femurs settle into the tibial plateau.
- The tibias nestle into the talus of the ankles.

The goal in Tadasana, as with the other standing poses, is to maintain this position relative to gravity. When we move in balance with gravity, our limbs, relative to each other, have balanced movement.

風

Live each season as it passes; breathe the air, drink the drink, taste the fruit and resign yourself to the influences of each.

— Source unknown

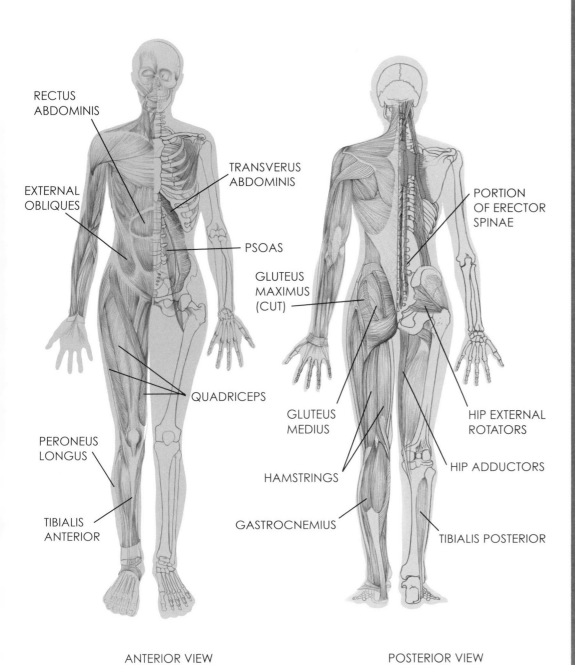

RECTUS
ABDOMINIS

TRANSVERUS
ABDOMINIS

EXTERNAL
OBLIQUES

PSOAS

PORTION
OF ERECTOR
SPINAE

GLUTEUS
MAXIMUS
(CUT)

QUADRICEPS

GLUTEUS
MEDIUS

HIP EXTERNAL
ROTATORS

PERONEUS
LONGUS

HAMSTRINGS

HIP ADDUCTORS

TIBIALIS
ANTERIOR

GASTROCNEMIUS

TIBIALIS POSTERIOR

ANTERIOR VIEW

POSTERIOR VIEW

Fig 4-1 Tadasana

Settling the femur heads into the acetabulum

A series of muscles helps stabilize the connection between the acetabulum of the pelvis and the femurs: the external rotators, the hip adductors, and the psoas.

The external rotators were first introduced in the principles of movement. Attaching to the greater trochanter, their role is to rotate the greater trochanter outward, toward the ischium. The hip adductors, attaching to the pelvis on both the pubis and ischium as well as to the femur, move the femur toward the midline of the body as well as rotate the femur slightly medially. The psoas, which will be explored later in this section, attaches to both the spine and the lesser trochanter of the femur. In this situation, acting as a hip flexor, it pulls the femur toward the body in hip flexion.

Together, these three muscle groups collectively settle the head of the femur into the acetabulum.

Settling the condyles of the femurs into the tibial plateau

The femur connects to the tibia at the knee joint by a series of muscles that originate in three distinct places – on the pelvis, from the shaft of the femur, and just above the knee joint. Primary support is provided by five groups of muscles:

- The quadriceps, which extends the leg at the knee
- The hamstrings, popliteus, plantaris, and gastrocnemius, all of which flex the leg at the knee; the popliteus allows for some lateral rotation at the knee as well

Together these muscles balance the structure of the femur and tibia at the knee.

Nestling the tibia into the saddle of the talus

Several muscles attach to the fibula or tibia as well as the foot to create stability of the ankle joint:

Muscle	Action on Ankle	Action on Foot
Tibialis anterior	Dorsiflexion	Inversion
Extensor hallucis longus	Dorsiflexion	Inversion
Extensor digitorum longus	Dorsiflexion	Eversion
Fibularis (peroneus) tertius	Dorsiflexion	Eversion
Fibularis (peroneus) longus & brevis	Plantar flexion	Eversion
Tibialis posterior	Plantar flexion	Inversion
Flexor hallucis longus	Plantar flexion	Inversion
Flexor digitorum longus	Plantar flexion	Inversion
Gastrocnemius and soleus	Plantar flexion	No direct action

If all this information overwhelms you, don't worry. Have a sip of water and take a breath. Standing poses have more going on than all of the other poses. The poses are simple when completed well, but to move into them safely and strongly requires us to unearth some of the interactions between muscle, fascia, and bone. The interactions will become clearer as we further explore our movement into other standing positions and as we delve into the injuries that tend to result when movement occurs too quickly or inappropriately.

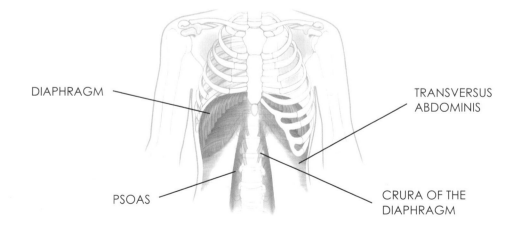

Fig 4-2 The diaphragm, its crura and the psoas

How the Upper Body Works in Standing Poses

Let's explore Tadasana (Mountain Pose) further – moving from the legs and pelvis up into the torso, head, and arms.

The action upward requires a few key elements:

- The pelvis connects with the spine.
- The spine connects with the rib cage.
- The spine and rib cage connect with the shoulder girdle and arms.
- The spine connects with the skull.

Connecting the pelvis with the spine

From section 3, principles of movement, we initially explored the concepts of connecting the spine with the pelvis. In Tadasana, there is one primary connection – the psoas. This may seem odd, since the psoas as a muscle doesn't directly connect with the pelvis; rather, it attaches on the femur and on the spine.

Let's look deeper:

The psoas muscle is a deep, strong muscle that cuddles into the lower half of the spine. It begins at the 12th thoracic vertebra, snuggles along each of the lumbar vertebrae, and attaches onto the femur at the lesser trochanter. It has been described as a muscle that stabilizes the spine, acting as a bridge between the legs and the torso. When working in balance with the leg muscles described earlier, the psoas gives a sense of grounding and centeredness to standing poses, and in turn, lightness to the spine.

Connecting the spine with the rib cage

The spine connects to the rib cage via the myofascial interactions between the psoas and diaphragm. Remember from section 3 that the diaphragm has two parts – the dome and the crura (fig 4-2). The crura make up the handle that attaches the diaphragm onto the lower thoracic and the first two or three lumbar vertebrae. Since part of the psoas attaches here as well, the fascia of each keep the connection moving upward.

Connecting the spine and rib cage with the shoulder girdle and arms

Since we explored the connections of the rib cage, shoulder girdle, and arms in inversions, back bends, and twists, we will take some time in this section to explore the connections between the rib cage and spine.

From the diaphragm, there are fascial connections with the lungs and the transversus thoracis. The lungs sit on the dome of the diaphragm. The transversus thoracis rests on the inside of the sternum, attaching from the sternum to the costal cartilage of the ribs. When it is tight the ribs depress, so when in Tadasana, some yogis will want to nurture it to release to help lift the ribs.

The pectoralis major is on the superficial side of the rib cage, attaching from the clavicle, sternum, and ribs onto the greater tubercle of the humerus. The pectoralis minor, as previously explored, attaches on the coracoid process of the scapula and onto the rib cage at the 3rd to 5th ribs. With the pectoralis major and minor tight, there is a tendency for a forward slump of the shoulder girdle, so as with the transversus thoracis, yoginis with this disposition will want to encourage it to release to help open the chest.

Connecting the spine with the skull

So far, the standing poses have gained grounding from the feet, through the legs, across the pelvis, onto the spine, and into the rib cage. From the rib cage back to the spine via the manubrium is the fascia of the infrahyoid muscles. The infrahyoid muscles help maintain structure of the junction between the cervical spine and the thoracic spine. They feed into the longus colli, longus capitis, rectus capitis anterior, and rectus capitis lateralis, all of which were introduced when jalandara bandha was explored in section 3.

Does T12 ring a bell?

There is a connection on the back side as well. From the diaphragm, across the rib cage, and into the cervical spine is the trapezius muscle. The trapezius attaches to the 7th cervical vertebra and all of the thoracic vertebrae, with its most inferior attachment at T12 *(fig 4-3)*.

T12 is the vertebra where the crura of the diaphragm and part of the psoas attach.

Is your curiosity piqued? Read on (to page 54), because this chain of muscles connects together to create balance, ease, and strength.

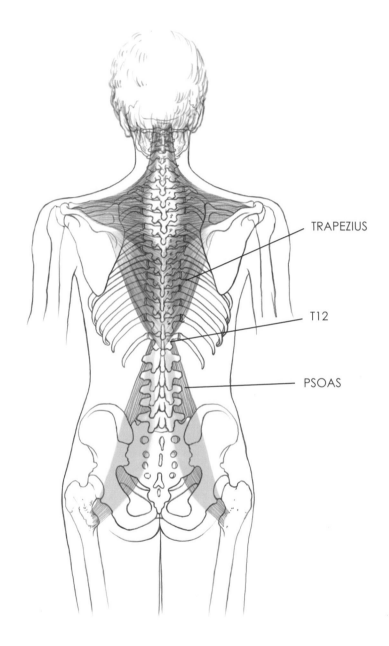

TRAPEZIUS

T12

PSOAS

Fig 4-3 A posterior view of the connection between the psoas and trapezius

 Deep flowing breath is essentially arousing and exciting.

— *Michael Sky*

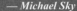

Back, Neck, and Knee Pain in Standing Poses

No matter if you are in Tadasana (Mountain Pose), moving into Utkatasana (Fierce/Powerful Pose), in Trikonasana (Triangle Pose), or in Virabhadrasana 1, 2, or 3 (Warrior 1, 2, or 3 Pose), there is potential for injuring the knees, lower back, or mid-back.

Why does this happen?

The tendency for injury in standing poses often occurs because of poor communication between the spine, pelvis, legs, and feet. There are three reasons for this:

1	2	3	
The combined movement between the femur, pelvis, and spine	**Foot support**	**General posture**	For these three reasons, standing poses can create problems in our bodies.
These three segments of the body are meant to work both independently and together in standing poses. When there is tightness or weakness within the segments on one side and between segments on both sides, dysfunctional movement occurs between the legs, pelvis, and spine. This leads to compensations that cause pain not only in the lower back and SI joint but also higher up in the mid-back and shoulder girdle or lower down in the knees and ankles.	The placement, flexibility, and resiliency of the feet will directly impact the ability of the energy in the body to rebound from the floor up through the legs and into the spine.	Kyphosis, or rounding of the thoracic spine, creates dysfunction between the shoulder girdle and rib cage, which impacts the ability of muscles to balance the lower spine as it relates to the pelvis. This imbalance can lead to problems further down the legs. Rounding of the spine will also affect the ability of the arms to move fully in all directions.	

How do I make my standing poses smooth yet powerful?

To create ease and power through the standing poses, follow the eight major principles of movement:

1. Nourish relaxation by breathing and connecting.
2. Initiate movement at the spine.
3. Connect spinal movement with moving through the largest joints first.
4. Move your joints through their optimum range of motion.
5. Create core stability by boosting up your bandhas and breathing.
6. Be relaxed and resilient.
7. Be generous with yourself and move through your pain-free range of motion.
8. Remember that less is more.

In addition to these eight principles of movement, explore the following four principles associated specifically with standing poses.

Principles Specific to Standing Poses

1. Relax

Relaxing in standing poses helps you develop awareness of the feet. When standing on one or both feet, you can feel the grounding action subtly move into the floor while simultaneously feeling the rebound of energy through the legs into the torso. This gives the yogi a chance to feel how the spine is responding, to feel what sensations exist, to feel the sense of strength, and to feel what is working and not working.

2. Begin with the Spine in Neutral

Tadasana (Mountain Pose) *(fig 4-4)* is a brilliant place to begin all standing poses because it gently inspires the body to lift upward to the sky, a movement that is quite opposite to the slouching position so common from working in front of computers.

A Closer Look at the Trapezius and Psoas

By cultivating a neutral position of the spine, the trapezius and psoas muscles can nurture their functional relationship. As stated earlier in this section, the trapezius muscle's inferior attachment is at T12, which is the same point of attachment for part of the crura of the diaphragm and the psoas.

Let's look deeper:

Consider that the trapezius also attaches to the 7th thoracic vertebra, each of the cervical vertebrae, and the scapula. The psoas attaches to each of the lumbar vertebrae, over the pelvis, and onto the femur at the lesser trochanter. The diaphragm rests inside the rib cage, attaching to the sternum and ribs and fascially connecting to the lungs and heart, while its crura attach to the first two or three lumbar vertebrae in addition to attaching to T12.

How the trapezius, diaphragm, and psoas interrelate can have a direct impact on how the standing pose is experienced – how the rib cage articulates with the spine and shoulder girdle, and how the spine articulates with the pelvis and legs. The leg positioning will directly affect the positioning of the feet.

A direct application with Tadasana (Mountain Pose)

In Tadasana, contract your upper trapezius muscles. Your scapulae will elevate toward your ears. Keep in mind that other neck muscles will be involved in this contraction – only for simplicity will we call it the action of the upper trapezius. Feel what happens to your breathing, the positioning of your lower spine, and the positioning of your legs right down into your feet. Now relax.

In Tadasana again, increase the lordosis, or arch, of your lower back. Be sure you are initiating the lordosis from your spine rather than initiating it by tilting your pelvis. Notice what happens to your breathing and to the positioning of your feet, legs, pelvis, and shoulder girdle.

3. Work from a Balanced Weight-Bearing Pelvis

A balanced weight-bearing pelvis refers to the pelvis when we are standing or when we are walking or running. The pelvis needs to be balanced in order for the upper body to transfer weight adequately to the lower body. If the weight transfer of the upper body – via the head, neck, rib cage, and spine – through the hip sockets, legs, knees, and feet is inadequate, compensations will occur to make up for the imbalance of the pelvis.

Balance comes from the interaction of several muscles working between the spine, rib cage, pelvis, and femurs:

- The rectus abdominis and obliques
- The quadratus lumborum
- The erector spinae
- The psoas
- The hip external rotators
- The hamstrings
- The quadriceps
- The hip abductors
- The hip adductors
- The muscles of the feet

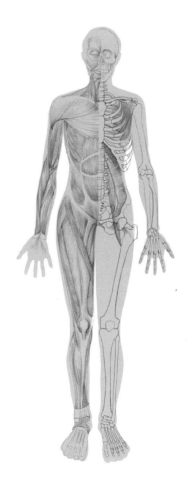

Fig 4-4 Tadasana (Mountain pose)

A direct application with Virabhadrasana 2 (Warrior 2 Pose)

Virabhadrasana 2 (Warrior 2 Pose) is a great asana to explore balance in the weight-bearing pelvis since one leg is in flexion while the other is in extension and external rotation.

From Tadasana (Mountain Pose), move into Virabhadrasana 2. As you are in the pose, notice if your front knee is moving toward the midline of your body or if you are experiencing any strain, any pain, or any other sensation in your lower or mid-back. If either is happening, chances are your pelvis isn't balanced.

Let's look further:

Knee Movement Inward in Virabhadrasana 2 (Warrior 2 Pose)

If the knee is moving toward the midline of the body, there tends to be imbalance between the hip abductors, external rotators, and hip adductors and the hip medial rotators. To check, move your pose against a wall. While in Virabhadrasana 2 (Warrior Pose 2), place a block between your front mid-thigh and the wall. Gently hold the block against the wall. Notice if your knee is now in line with the second toe of the front foot.

For fun, move from Virabhadrasana 2 (Warrior 2 Pose) into Utthita Parsvakonasana (Extended Side Angle Pose). Be sure you keep the block between your front mid-thigh and the wall. Do you feel the block slipping? If you do, just bring it back into position.

Depending on who you are and what your body is experiencing, you will feel this position slightly differently. Some people feel this as a muscle contraction in their hip abductors or external rotators; others feel it as a release in the hip adductors, or even as a combination of both. Whichever your experience, you are strengthening the balance of your pelvis.

Lower Back Pain in Virabhadrasana 2 (Warrior 2 Pose)

Let's address the back leg in this pose. Sometimes the positioning of the back leg leads to problems in the SI joint, lower back, and mid-back.

In Virabhadrasana 2 (Warrior 2 Pose) (fig 4-5), the back leg is straight, in extension and external rotation. Sometimes in this position, back pain occurs in the area of the SI joint, in the lower lumbar spine, or even midway up.

Why does this happen?

The key to the position is the combination of external rotation and extension of the back leg while the front leg is in flexion. However, sometimes the pure combined movement of external rotation and extension does not occur at the hip socket. Instead, a jamming feeling occurs in the SI joint area, lower back, or mid-back. To help remedy this, shift the relationship between the back leg and the pelvis.

How do I do this?

If the right leg is back, step the right leg out to the right slightly. Notice if there is any strain or jamming in the lower back or SI joint. If strain continues, move the foot and leg a little further to the right, until pain no longer occurs. This works because it gives your hips more freedom for movement. Your alignment won't be perfect according to some systems of yoga; however, as your hips release and regain balance, you will be back in traditional alignment before you know it.

4. Feel Your Feet as Firm and Supple

Firmness and suppleness are often best described in images. In the feet, firmness is like a pyramid. Strong and stable, its inherent structure gives a sense of grounding. Suppleness is movement – a fluid rebound-

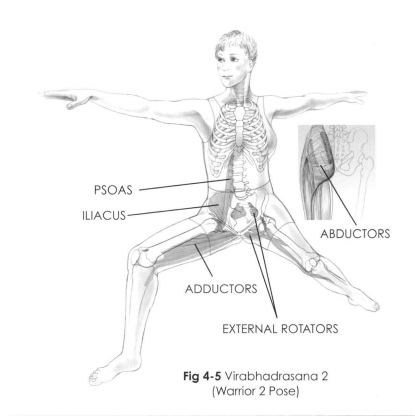

PSOAS
ILIACUS
ABDUCTORS
ADDUCTORS
EXTERNAL ROTATORS

Fig 4-5 Virabhadrasana 2 (Warrior 2 Pose)

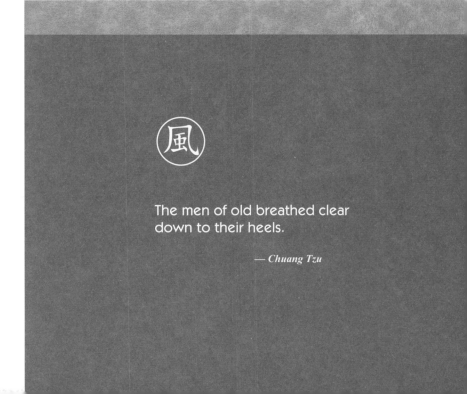

風

The men of old breathed clear down to their heels.

— *Chuang Tzu*

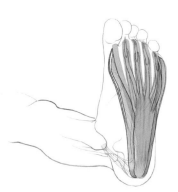

Fig 4-6 Plantar fascia

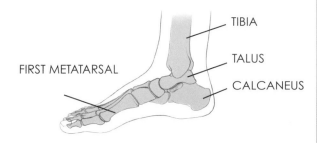

TIBIA

FIRST METATARSAL

TALUS

CALCANEUS

Fig 4-7 Medial view of foot

ing effect that generates propulsion or shock absorption. Together, firmness and suppleness bring resiliency, the ability to bear the body's weight while simultaneously feeling the energy of the floor below.

Firmness: A Closer Look at the Pyramid

The pyramid of the foot begins at the talus, a bone that, from above, is shaped like a saddle. Nestled inside the saddle is the tibia. It is at this articulation that the foot receives the body's weight (fig 4-7).

From the talus, the foot spans out to three points that form the base of the pyramid. The first point, radiating backward and downward, is the centre of the calcaneus (the heel bone). The second point is at the head of the first metatarsal (the ball of the foot). The third point is at the head of the fifth metatarsal (the base of the pinky toe).

Applying anatomy to asanas: The arches of the feet

Take some time to explore your feet, feeling the three points and the spaces between the points. Are you holding your feet with hardness, or is the lift through the arches of the feet happening with effortless effort, with a sense of nourishing ease? Bring your awareness to the bottom of your feet. Feel your feet touching the floor or your yoga mat. Feel where the metatarsals join with the phalanges (the toes). Become aware of the calcaneus (the heel bone). Notice how the talus interacts with the tibia to form your ankle joint. How balanced does it feel? Now move into Vrksasana (Tree Pose). Notice how each foot is feeling and how they are contributing to your practice – are you holding your feet with hardness, or is the lift through the arches of the feet happening with effortless effort, with a sense of nourishing ease?

Suppleness: A Closer Look at the Arches of the Feet

Imagine you have just stepped out of the water and are standing on a wooden dock. You take a few steps and look behind. You see the imprint of your wet feet on the dry dock. If you have a "normal" foot, you won't see the full bottom side of your foot in that footprint; instead you will see only the toes, the lateral edge of the foot, the ball of the foot, and the heel. These are the elements of the pyramid. What you don't see are the elements of the arches.

There are three arches of the foot that together act as shock absorbers. They support the weight of the body when we are standing still in Tadasana (Mountain Pose) and bring about propulsion when moving into Virabhadrasana 3 (Warrior 3 Pose). Two of the three arches originate at the calcaneus and run forward toward the toes. Because of their direction, we call them "longitudinal" arches. The longi

tudinal arch that runs from the calcaneus to the head of the first metatarsal is the medial longitudinal arch; the longitudinal arch that runs from the calcaneus to the head of the fifth metatarsal is the lateral longitudinal arch. The third arch is the transverse arch, which connects the two longitudinal arches at the forefoot.

Sustaining the Feet: The Muscles and Fascia

Sustenance is nourishment, and for the feet, sustenance comes from the muscles and fascia. When muscles and fascia lose their normal functional pattern, they can shift the mechanics of the feet entirely, causing and irritating all sorts of conditions, from fallen arches, bunions, and heel spurs to pronation and supination. Muscles and fascia are essential elements to support the firmness and the suppleness the feet naturally have.

Sustaining the arches with effortless effort and nourishing ease comes from the interaction of muscles and fascia. When the interaction of the muscles and fascia is functional, we are more able to feel the two-way energy exchange between us and the earth. From us, our energy can seep into the earth and spread like roots in soil. From the earth, we can feel the return of energy back into our feet and through our bodies.

The Key Players

We have already introduced the tibialis posterior and the fibularis (peroneus) longus in a few other sections of the book. So in this section our focus will be the muscles on the base of the foot and the plantar fascia (fig 4-6).

Muscular support from below

Sitting on the floor or on a chair, place one foot on your knee. Turn the bottom, or sole, of your foot over so that you can look at it. Take one finger and place it on your calcaneus, in the center of the heel. Draw a diagonal line toward your big toe. That is the medial longitudinal arch. Now take your finger back to the center of your heel. Draw a diagonal line toward your pinky toe. That is the lateral longitudinal arch.

The key muscles that support these arches are the flexor hallucis longus and the abductor hallucis on the medial arch and the abductor digiti minimi on the lateral arch. The flexor digitorum brevis and the quadratus plantae support both longitudinal arches.

While still sitting, place your foot on the floor, sole touching the floor. About one third of the way between your ankle and toes is the transverse arch, which connects the two longitudinal arches. The primary muscle that supports the transverse arch is the adductor hallucis.

Plantar fascia – The fascial support of the arches

Surrounding and threading through the musculature of the feet are bands of fascia. The largest, most superficial, and best known is the plantar fascia, which spans most of the foot, from the calcaneus to the top of the metatarsals (not into the toes). When we press weight into our feet in yoga asanas, the ball of the foot and the heel want to spread away from each other. The plantar fascia helps contain and maintain the organization of the muscles so that the arches stay intact.

Applying anatomy to asanas: Softening "hard" feet

The analogy "hard" feet is appropriate since so many students seem to have lost the fluidity of their feet. Toes have clenched, arches have "dropped," or bunions have grown. It is as if they are standing in concrete, unable to feel or move energy from the earth through the feet. A great way to bring aliveness back into the feet is to take a tennis or similar type ball and roll it under each foot for two minutes. Then, have a seat on the floor and roll out your calf muscle – the back side of the calf (gastrocnemius muscle) and the outside, where the fibularis (peroneus) longus is located. Then come back into Tadasana and feel what is there....

back bends

Back bends are delicious.

They release the muscles and connective tissue on the front of the body and strengthen the muscles on the back of the body. They provide a sense of elegance and efficiency to improving posture and to revitalizing energy flow. Some would say that back bends far exceed caffeine's kick-start by instead providing a calm way to tame the sagging slump that can overcome a busy mind. Although back bends provide many benefits, there are also some risks to performing them. A common problem that arises for people practicing back bends is "jamming of the back," which leads to lower back, mid-back, and/or neck pain. This pain can lead to biomechanical dysfunction of the shoulder and pelvic girdles, possibly leading to referred pain and dysfunction down the arms and legs, respectively. So it is important to begin by relaxing first and *then* moving – and when you do initiate movement, begin with the spine in mind.

In my time in India, I experienced back bends in a completely different way. In India, programs of back bends are designed for people suffering from cardiovascular disease. The theory is that back bends enable the release of the muscles and fascia of the chest, between the ribs, and particularly of the pericardium (the membrane that envelops the heart). This allows more space for the heart, improving its functioning. While published data does not exist on the effectiveness or truth of this theory, the anecdotal stories and the positive changes in the students' ECGs (electrocardiograms) certainly captivate the curiosity about the effects of back bends on our health and healing.

Back Bends and the Spine

The spine is the central channel of movement in all poses and particularly in back bends because of its specific role of moving into extension. Without spinal extension there would be no back bend.

Begin with the Spine in Mind: Moving with Gravity and Moving against Gravity

Glancing in any yoga book, you will notice that all back bends can be classified into one of two groups: back bends that move with gravity, called traction back bends, and back bends that move against gravity, called contraction back bends.[1]

Let's take a look:

Traction back bends move with gravity. Typically, they begin from kneeling or from standing; however, they also occur over chairs, bolsters, and blocks. To move into the pose, the body needs to fall with gravity toward the floor. Examples of traction back bends are Supta Baddha Konasana (Reclining Bound Angle Pose), Ustrasana (Camel Pose) *(fig 4-8)*, and Urdhva Dhanurasana from Tadasana (Upward Bow Pose, Back Bend, or Wheel from Standing).

Contraction back bends move against gravity. Typically, they begin from a prone position, with the belly to the floor. To move into the pose, the body needs to lift up and away from the floor. Examples of contraction back bends are Bhujangasana (Cobra Pose), Salabhasana (Locust Pose), and Dhanurasana (Bow Pose) (fig 4-9).

Both groups of back bends require the spine to move into extension, so they require the same primary muscles to contract and release. However, because of the different relationship with gravity, each type of back bend requires a different quality of muscular action to stabilize and support in order to maintain control and smoothness throughout the movement.

Let's explore further:

Traction back bends initially require control and then release of the muscles on the front of the body to keep the movement with gravity smooth and paced. Control comes in the form of eccentric contractions of the rectus abdominis, psoas, obliques (bilaterally), and pectoralis major and minor. In some poses, the rectus femoris (one of the quadriceps muscles) will also contribute eccentric control. Once control and smoothness are created, traction back bends then require these same muscles to release, enabling a deeper experience of the pose.

Contraction back bends require more strength of the back muscles, primarily the erector spinae, to overcome the pull of gravity. For more complex poses, the lower trapezius and the mid to lower fibers of the latissimus dorsi contract to help support the extension of the spine that was initiated by the erector spinae. As well, contractions of the gluteus maximus, a powerful extensor of the hip, and the hamstrings are utilized to help lift the legs in positions such as Dvipada Salabhasana (Two Feet up in Locust) and full Dhanurasana (Bow Pose).

Traction Back Bends	Contraction Back Bends
Move with gravity	**Move against gravity**
Require muscles on front of body to eccentrically contract to control movement with gravity and then release to move deeper into the pose	Require back muscles to concentrically contract to overcome gravity
Primary muscles eccentrically contracting: rectus abdominis, psoas, obliques (bilaterally), pectoralis major and minor, rectus femoris (in some poses)	Primary muscles concentrically contracting: erector spinae Lower trapezius indirectly supports the extension of the spine by drawing the shoulder blades down the back

Contraction back bends move against gravity. Typically, they begin from a prone position, with the belly to the floor.

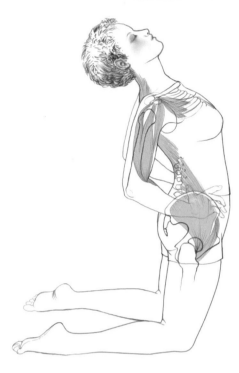

Fig 4-8 Traction back bend:
Ustrasana (Camel Pose)

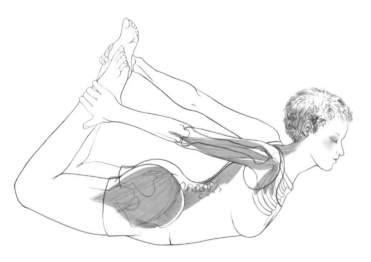

Fig 4-9 Contraction back bend:
Dhanurasana (Bow Pose)

Jamming of the Spine: The Path of Least Resistance

No matter if you are moving into a traction or contraction back bend, the same primary risk needs to be addressed – moving through the path of least resistance causes jamming of the lower back.

Why does this happen?

The tendency to jam the lower back in back bends is an honest one. In fact, one could say that we are almost designed to jam the lower back.

How so?

Anatomically, extension is greater in the cervical and lumbar portions of the spine than in the thoracic spine. There are three reasons for this:

1

Structure of the vertebrae

The thoracic vertebrae have much longer spinous processes than those of the lumbar or cervical spine, so the thoracic vertebrae don't have the same range of motion.

2

The ribs attach to the thoracic vertebrae

In addition to vertebrae, the thoracic curve also contends with any tightness or deviation of the muscles attaching to the ribs themselves, which can also limit extension.

3

General posture

Since many people work in front of computers, most human posture has some kyphosis, or forward rounding of the thoracic spine. This causes the postural muscles of the thoracic spine to become tight or weak, which limits the thoracic spine extending backward.

For these three reasons, there is a tendency to move in the places that are easiest – the places with least resistance and with the least amount of stability and support. They are L5–S1, T12–L1, and C7–T1.

How do I make the curve smoother and safer so that my back doesn't jam?

To prevent jamming and to ensure smooth and easy movement, follow the eight major principles of movement:

1. Nourish relaxation by breathing and connecting.
2. Initiate movement at the spine.
3. Connect spinal movement with moving through the largest joints first.
4. Move your joints through their optimum range of motion.
5. Create core stability by boosting up your bandhas and breathing.
6. Be relaxed and resilient.
7. Be generous with yourself and move through your pain-free range of motion.
8. Remember that less is more.

In addition to these eight principles of movement, explore the five principles associated specifically with back bends.

Principles Specific to Back Bends

1. Relax

Because it is easy to complete a back bend by moving through the weak links of the spine, it is easy to create injury and dysfunction. So, to safely inspire a functional and balanced body, it is important to cultivate awareness of movement.

Breathe and relax before moving into any back bend. Being relaxed heightens awareness and encourages tighter, tenser areas of the body to release and let go, while also allowing for inner cues of what is working and what is not working to surface.

As the movement continues into the back bend, you may notice that you are particularly tight in one area of your spine or at your hips. As a result, full extension may not be possible. By being aware, you can prevent yourself from forcing through this and instead cultivate a different way of moving that enables release, stability, and strength.

2. Initiate Extension at the Thoracic Spine

Back bends provide a lovely laboratory for enjoying the spine in its full splendour. As mentioned earlier, in order to experience a back bend, the spine must extend. Without spinal extension, the back bend will not occur.

To optimize spinal extension, begin at the thoracic spine. By moving first at the thoracic spine, then maintaining the depth of the pose relative to the movement occurring at the thoracic spine, you are almost guaranteed to not overcompensate, which means you won't move through the weak links, which in turn means you won't jam the lower back and cause back or neck pain.

Applying anatomy to asana: Imagine that you can breathe into your sternum, and just your sternum; from the lungs outward. As your soft breath fills into the sternum, the rib cage gently lifts, as if of its own accord. The throat softens and the thoracic spine gently extends.

Why begin at the thoracic spine?

Initiating extension at the thoracic spine causes the following to happen:

1. The erector spinae muscles are directly engaged.
2. The lower trapezius muscles, which provide support to extension subsequent to the erector spinae contracting, are also engaged.

By engaging these groups of muscles, support is given to each segment of the spine, preventing a spinal collapse.

If you own or have access to Erich Schiffman's book *Moving into Stillness*, open it up and take a look at how he moves through his spine. His arch is much like the arch of a bridge – strong, smooth, fluid, round. He is not moving by using the hypermobile areas of C7–T1, T12–L1, and L5–S1. Instead, he is strong and stable throughout.

3. Release the Chest and Use the Back of the Shoulders

Sometimes initiating movement at the thoracic spine is difficult because the muscles of the chest are tight or desensitized. If the scapulae have the tendency to ride up to the ears, and the shoulders round forward, it can be difficult to access the segmental movement of the individual vertebrae of the thoracic spine.

How do I do this?

Follow these steps to release the chest, stabilize the scapulae, and use the back of the shoulders:

1. Release the pectoralis minor, coraco-brachialis, and biceps brachii.
2. Strengthen the connection of the rhomboids, teres minor, infraspinatus, and posterior deltoid.
3. Balance the rhomboids with the serratus anterior, levator scapulae, pectoralis minor, and lower trapezius.

A direct application with Dhanurasana (Bow Pose)

In asanas such as Dhanurasana (Bow Pose) *(fig 4-10)*, both mobility and strength of the arms can enable smooth and fluid movement.

In Dhanurasana, the arms are in extension in order to grasp the ankles. Strong and smooth extension of the humerus in the shoulder socket relies on the stability of the scapula. Stability of the scapula relies on muscles that attach directly to the spine. If those muscles aren't working functionally, the relationship between the spine, scapula, and humerus will also be dysfunctional, creating the possibility of moving through the weak links of the spine.

Let's take a look:

For the arm to move into extension, the humerus at the scapula must move into extension. For the humerus to move in this way, the scapula must be stabilized. The scapula is stabilized by the levator

scapulae, rhomboids, lower trapezius in the back, serratus anterior at the side, and pectoralis minor in the front. If the pectoralis minor is tight, the scapula will have the tendency to rise and rotate anteriorly. This position is unstable and will prevent the humerus from extending backward. So, in order to complete the pose, students typically roll the shoulders forward, which prevents extension through the thoracic spine. Without extension of the thoracic spine, there will be an automatic subconscious tendency to tilt the head back by hinging at C7–T1, to stick the ribs out by hinging at T12–L1, or to jam through the lower back by hinging at L5–S1 just to complete the movement.

4. Stabilize the Connection between the Pelvis and Spine and between the Pelvis and Femurs

Sometimes initiating movement at the thoracic spine and releasing the chest are difficult because the muscles of the lower back are tight, desensitized, or hypermobile. When the lower back is dysfunctional, there is a tendency for the pelvis to move with dysfunction as well. It can become stuck or unstable. Whichever the situation, both can lead to poor spinal movement, increasing the potential for pain and injury in the lower and mid-back. By improving the connection between the pelvis and spine and between the pelvis and femurs, you can gain a foundational structure from which your back bend can move safely and easily.

How do I do this?

Follow these steps to stabilize the pelvis:

1. Balance the action and activation of the transversus abdominis, obliques, multifidi, hip adductors, and anterior pelvic floor muscles.
2. Connect the action of the hamstrings, gluteus maximus, and lumbar spine with the balance of the hip rotators.

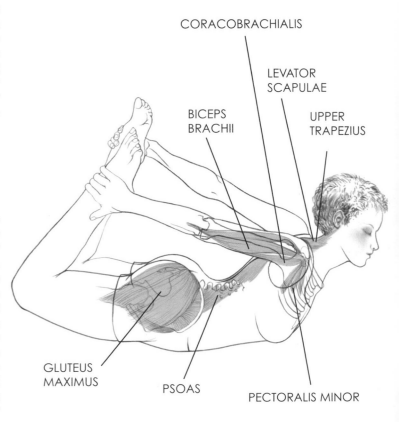

CORACOBRACHIALIS

LEVATOR SCAPULAE

BICEPS BRACHII

UPPER TRAPEZIUS

GLUTEUS MAXIMUS

PSOAS

PECTORALIS MINOR

Fig 4-10 Dhanurasana (Bow Pose)
(hamstrings are not shown in this drawing)

A direct application with Dhanurasana (Bow Pose)

Dhanurasana (Bow Pose) provides a laboratory for exploring pelvic girdle and leg movements as they relate to the spine. Specific to Dhanurasana, like all back bends that raise the legs off the floor, strong leg energy is required. Strong leg energy emerges from a stable pelvis.

Let's take a look:

Pelvic Stability: Transversus Abdominis, Obliques, Multifidi, Hip Adductors, Anterior Pelvic Floor

The pelvis remains stable by gently contracting the anterior portion of the pelvic floor, the transversus abdominis, internal obliques, and multifidi, along with the hip adductors. If any of these muscles are weak, if the contraction is unbalanced, or if the muscles are contracted with too much force and without breath, the foundational stability of the pelvis will be compromised, causing the legs to move weakly and the junction of the pelvis on the lumbar spine at L5–S1 to compensate. This can create dysfunctional movement, possible pain, and potential injury.

Leg Energy: Connecting the Hamstrings, Gluteus Maximus, and Lower Back with the Hip Rotators

For the legs to move into extension, the femurs must move into extension at the hip joints. For femurs to move in this way, the pelvis must remain stable.

From an anchored pelvis, the gluteus maximus and hamstrings contract, causing the femurs to lift into extension.

However, for yogis and yoginis with tight external rotators, this pure movement of hip extension is not possible. Tight external rotators

cause the femurs to roll outward. You will see this in Dhanurasana by looking at the entire leg and heel. The femurs, tibias, and heels will be turned toward each other. If leg extension was to occur in this position, the chances for pain in the lower back or around the SI joint would be higher than if the legs were not externally rotated.

So what to do?

Fan outward the stability gained in your pelvis. Read on....

5. Fan the Pelvic Stability Outward: Developing Your Core

Fanning the pelvic stability outward is the essence of developing solid core stability. Beginning at the pelvis and radiating up the spine and down to the toes, it is necessary if you want to experience strength, ease, lightness, depth, and freedom in a back bend – when performing traction back bends you will more readily experience a release of the muscles along the front of the body, while in contraction back bends you will feel a more dynamic lift upward.

Since we explored the chest and rib cage earlier in this section, our focus for fanning stability will be on the lower body.

Fanning Core Stability Downward

To fan stability downward, the foundational stability of the pelvis moves into the legs. The stabilizing action of the transversus abdominis, multifidi, and internal obliques, along with the contraction of the anterior pelvic floor muscles, moves into the hip adductors.

From the hip adductors, the core stabilizing energy moves into the feet, where it connects with the muscles of pada bandha. Pada bandha was introduced in principle 5 on page 40. Two of the muscles that create

pada bandha are the fibularis (peroneus) longus and tibialis posterior.

How do the hip adductors and pada bandha work in this situation?

The tibialis posterior and fibularis (peroneus) longus are functionally linked to the hip adductors. From the pelvis, the hip adductors gently pull the legs together with a slight internal rotation. If these muscles weren't opposed, the femurs would continue to rotate inward, creating an inner spiral right to the bottom of the feet. Instead, the fibularis (peroneus) longus and tibialis posterior anchor the foot and ankle, countering the inner rotation of the femurs. The arches lift and energy rebounds up the legs back into the core.

The breath becomes a stone; the stone, a plant; the plant, an animal; the animal, a man; the man, a spirit; and the spirit, a god.

— *Christian Nevell Bovee*

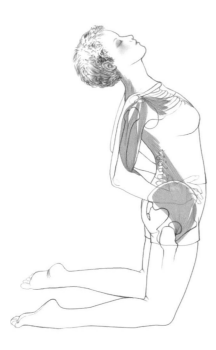

Fig 4-11 Ustrasana (Camel Pose)

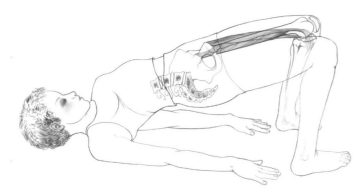

Fig 4-12 Setu Bandha Sarvangasana (Little Bridge Pose)

A direct application with Ustrasana (Camel Pose)

Prepare for Ustrasana (Camel Pose) *(fig 4-11)* from kneeling. Move into the asana. Gently ease out. Now, place two pressed foam blocks between your thighs, close to the pelvis. Be sure they are not touching the knees. Gently press the blocks together. When you do, you are using the hip adductors. Now move back into Ustrasana. Is there a difference? You probably noticed one or more of the following:

- A greater release of the muscles in the front of the body
- A deeper experience backward
- Less back pain

This experience can be used with any back bend.

A direct application with Setu Bandha Sarvangasana (Little Bridge Pose)

Prepare for Setu Bandha Sarvangasana (Little Bridge Pose) *(fig 4-12)* on your back with your knees bent. Move into the asana. Gently ease out. Now, place two pressed foam blocks between your thighs, close to the pelvis. Be sure they are not touching the knees. Gently press the blocks together. When you do, you are using the hip adductors. Now move back into Setu Bandha Sarvangasana. Is there a difference?

Come out of the pose. Now place your attention on your feet – specifically, the center of your heel, the ball of your foot, and the base of your pinky toe. Now move back into the pose. What do you feel? Is there a difference? Now, combine the two – hip adductors and feet. Any difference?

To Contract or Not Contract Your Butt

This is a common question and point of discussion for a back bending practice. Some teachers suggest utilizing the gluteus maximus muscles to create a posterior pelvic tilt, or pelvic tuck, which lengthens the lower back and creates space. The idea is to lengthen the back to prevent jamming. Other teachers suggest relaxing the gluteus maximus muscle.

The answer lies in the stability generated in the pelvis and how that stability can transform into strength, ease, and freedom.

What happens when we tuck the pelvis?

When we tuck the pelvis, the pelvis itself rotates posteriorly. If we are lying supine, on our backs, the lower back will also flatten to the floor. The pubic bone lifts toward the navel. As a result the primary muscle engaged is the rectus abdominis.

The question is, does this muscle contribute to stability and ease of movement?

To determine if a muscle contributes to stability of the spine, we need to look at the muscles that connect directly to the spine. The rectus abdominis, being the most superficial muscle of the abdominal muscle group, is quite distant from the spinal vertebrae. Because of its distance, it cannot have direct influence on lumbar stability. As a result this position does not contribute to stability and, as such, does not protect the lower back from injury.

So what to do?

Utilize the pelvic and lumbar stabilizers, the hip adductors, and pada bandha. Work toward releasing the chest and softening the throat; your tendencies to move through the weak links will minimize and your strength, power, and ease will maximize.

If you don't have blocks handy, imagine that the heads of your femurs are moving together; or imagine that you are holding a ball between your thighs. Be sure that it is near the upper thigh and not between the knees. By accessing the spot closest to your pelvis, you are activating a greater percentage of the adductors.

forward bends

Forward bends are gracious.

Where back bends are delicious, forward bends are gracious. They require us to be patient, gentle, and quiet as the tightness that occupies the back side of the body unravels, lets go, and releases. As the tightness releases, the whole back side becomes stronger.

Where back bends are delicious, forward bends are gracious. They require us to be patient, gentle, and quiet as the tightness that occupies the back side of the body unravels, lets go, and releases. As the tightness releases, the whole back side becomes stronger.

The release. In no other group of asanas do we rely so much on such a release to occur – the release of the plantar fascia, gastrocnemius, soleus, hamstrings, hip rotators, and erector spinae. This chain of muscles is the nemesis of many yoga practitioners when performing forward bends. Stories are told of people tearing hamstrings when an overzealous intention takes the forward bend deeper than the physical body can handle.

For this reason, the most important caution lies in what happens when ambition overrides patience. When ambition overrides patience, there is a tendency for the arms to pull the body further forward or to impose flexion on the spine earlier than necessary. Both put strain on the lower spine, SI joint, and hamstring attachments at the pelvic bones, tibia, and fibula. This strain can lead to spinal, hip, or knee dysfunction, which in turn leads to back or neck pain. So it is important to begin by relaxing first and *then* moving – and when you do initiate movement, begin by connecting spinal movement with the movement at the hip sockets.

Forward Bends, the Spine, and the Hip Sockets

Forward bends require two things to happen.

- To initiate the movement, forward flexion must occur at the hip sockets.
- For some forward bends, to deepen the movement, forward flexion continues through the spine.

Begin with the Spine in Mind: Be Sure to Move at the Hip Sockets

Forward bends provide telling evidence of the function of the hip sockets. There is a tendency for people who are tight in the hip sockets to overcompensate in forward bends by over-rounding the spine. They also have a tendency to feel a pain or strain in the lower back as they move further forward. Tight hip sockets also tend to lead to tight calf muscles, which further limits movement into a forward bend.

For all yogis, and especially yogis with tight hips, initiating movement at the hip sockets while maintaining a neutral spine helps create a connection between the spine and the hip, instilling better functioning of the femur-pelvis-spine complex and the femur-tibia-ankle-foot complex.

Forward Bends and Gravity: Moving with Gravity and Moving Against Gravity

As with back bends, there are forward bends that move with gravity and forward bends that move against gravity.

Let's take a look:

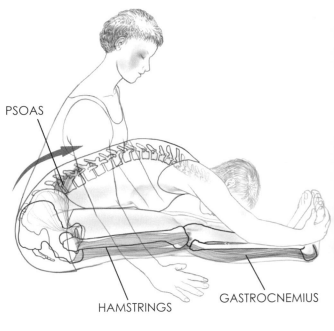

PSOAS

HAMSTRINGS

GASTROCNEMIUS

Fig 4-13 Paschimottanasana (Sitting Forward Fold)

1

Standing forward bends

Standing forward bends all move with gravity. Examples of standing forward bends are Uttanasana (Standing Forward Bend) (fig 4-14), Parsvottanasana (Pyramid Pose), and Prasarita Padottanasana (Wide-Legged Forward Bend) (fig 4-15).

2

Sitting forward bends

Sitting forward bends move with gravity; however, compared with standing forward bends, gravity has less impact. Examples of sitting forward bends are Supta Parvatasana (Forward Fold in Lotus with Hands above Head), Paschimottanasana (Intense West Stretch/Sitting Forward Fold) (fig 4-13), and Janu Sirsasana (Head to Knee Pose/Modified Runner's Stretch).

3

Supine forward bends

Supine forward bends move against gravity. Examples of supine forward bends are Supta Padangusthasana (Supine Hamstring Stretch) (fig 4-18) and Urdhva Prasarita Padasana (Upward Extended Feet Pose).

All three groups of forward bends require the spine to initially be in neutral while the femurs and pelvis move – either the femurs move while the pelvis stays quiet to bring the leg(s) closer to the torso or the pelvis moves and the femurs remain quiet to bring the torso closer to the leg(s). While both standing and sitting forward bends require some spinal flexion near the end range of movement into the asana, all three groups of forward bends have their primary movement at the hip sockets. Because of this similarity, the same muscles will contract and release for all three types of forward bends. However, because of the different relationship with gravity, and the different relationship between the limbs in some asanas, each type of forward bend will have a slightly different focus to experience depth while building strength, enabling release, and maintaining smooth control.

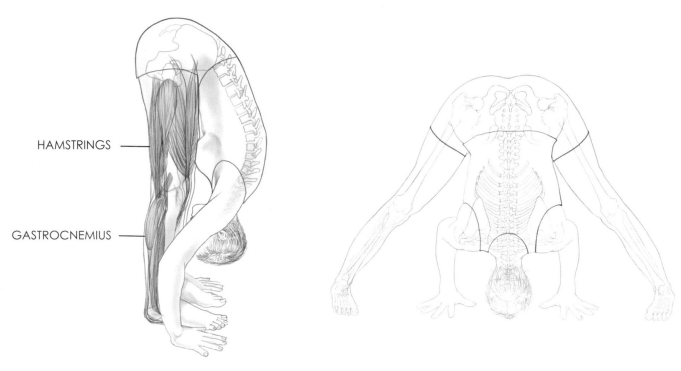

HAMSTRINGS

GASTROCNEMIUS

Fig 4-14 Uttanasana (Standing Forward Bend)

Fig 4-15 Prasarita Padottanasana (Wide-Legged Forward Bend)

In standing forward bends … gravity is the primary cause of the movement, and the muscles that are the most well known for creating flexion at the hip joint, the psoas and iliacus, are only contracting passively.

Let's explore further:

Standing Forward Bends

Standing forward bends have the smallest base of support. This base is constructed with the feet and either has both feet close together, side by side as in Uttanasana (Standing Forward Bend) (fig 4-14); apart, one behind the other as in Parsvottanasana (Pyramid Pose); or apart and side by side as in Prasarita Padottanasana (Wide-Legged Forward Bend) (fig 4-15).

With each of these asanas, gravity accelerates the movement forward and downward. In fact, gravity is the primary cause of the movement, and the muscles that are the most well known for creating flexion at the hip joint, the psoas and iliacus, are only contracting passively. Since gravity is the primary force moving the body downward, the extensors – such as the erector spinae, hamstrings, and some of the fibers of their partner muscles, the gastrocnemius and hip rotators – must contract eccentrically to control the descent downward while helping to maintain the head of the femur in the hip socket. Since they are contracting to do this, there is less willingness for these muscles to release and "let go," compared with forward bends that occur in sitting or supine positions.

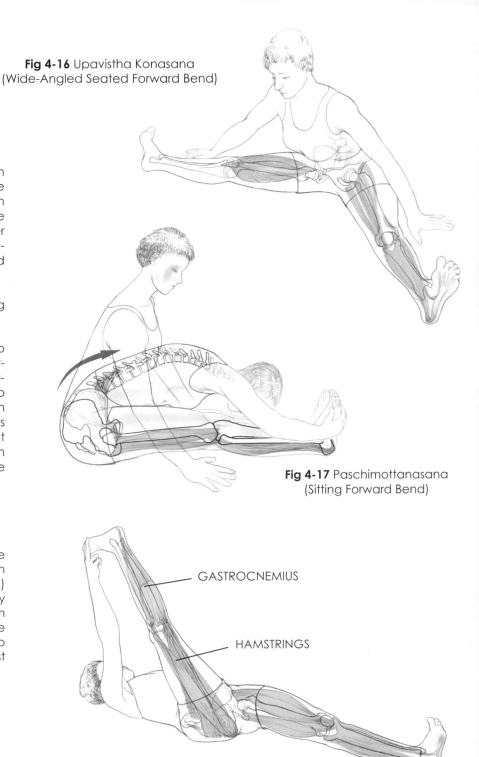

Fig 4-16 Upavistha Konasana
(Wide-Angled Seated Forward Bend)

Sitting Forward Bends

Sitting forward bends have a larger base of support than standing forward bends. In addition to having the ischial tuberosities on the floor (or on a block on the floor), the legs are crossed in a lotus position as in Supta Parvatasana (Forward Fold in Lotus with Hands above Head); the legs are outstretched as in Paschimottanasana (Intense West Stretch/Sitting Forward Fold) *(fig 4-17)*; one leg is outstretched while the other leg is in a different position as in Janu Sirsasana (Head to Knee Pose/Modified Runner's Stretch); or with both legs spread wide as in Upavistha Konasana (Wide-Angled Forward Bend) *(fig 4-16)*.

Gravity has an effect on sitting forward bends, but not to the extent as in standing forward bends, where the legs are required to keep you upright.

The greater effect on sitting forward bends is the positioning of the legs relative to each another. In most bodies, when the legs are both outstretched as in Paschimottanasana (Intense West Stretch/Sitting Forward Fold) *or apart as in Upanstha Konasana (Wide-Angled Forward Bend) (fig 4-16)*, both sides of the pelvis are moving into flexion. The same movement is happening on both sides of the body. In positions such as Janu Sirsasana (Head to Knee Pose/Modified Runner's Stretch), where one leg is outstretched and the other is flexed at the hip and knee and externally rotated at the hip, the same thing is not happening on both sides. This situation can lead to an imbalanced sitting position and can limit the degree of flexion available through the hip sockets.

Fig 4-17 Paschimottanasana
(Sitting Forward Bend)

Supine Forward Bends

Supine forward bends have the largest base of support. All of these asanas require you to be on your back. Either one or both legs are pointed toward the ceiling. With these forward bends, such as Supta Padangusthasana (Supine Hamstring Stretch) *(fig 4-18)*, the legs are not required to support your body's weight, nor are they moving with gravity. As well, since the back is on the floor, with the pelvis and sacrum in neutral, the erector spinae are also not involved in the movement. Therefore, the movement is one of pure hip flexion, with the heads of the femurs moving in the hip sockets, giving the hamstrings (and, if the knees are straight, gastrocnemius) the best opportunity for a true release.

GASTROCNEMIUS

HAMSTRINGS

Fig 4-18 Supta Padangusthasana
(Supine Hamstring Stretch)

Tearing, Pulling, and Injuring the Hamstrings and Back

The action of tearing, pulling, and injuring the hamstrings and lower back occurs mostly as a result of going too far, too fast in standing and sitting forward bends.

Why does this happen?

1

Gravity

Gravity imposes a number of difficult or complex scenarios in yoga. Because it accelerates the body's movement toward the earth, without proper support and stability a body could get injured. As it relates to forward bends, its influence has created cautionary red flags warning people to move carefully so that they prevent damage to the back, injury to a disc, or strain anywhere from the bottom of the feet to the base of the skull.

2

Leveraging with the arms too soon

Whether you are moving into standing, sitting, or supine forward bends, using the arms to leverage the body forward further before the hips have reached the end of their safe range of motion will create greater spinal flexion as opposed to greater movement in the hip sockets. This can damage the integrity of the spinal discs and injure the hamstring tendons, sacroiliac ligaments, and thoracolumbar fascia.

3

Ironclad hamstrings and tight hips

Movement forward requires movement in the hip sockets. The muscles directly associated with the movement of the femur in the acetabulum of the pelvis are the hip and hamstring muscles. When these muscles are tight, movement forward will be limited.

4

Tight connective tissue

While forward bends rely on movement through the hip sockets either by the femurs moving toward the torso or the pelvis moving toward the legs, influences beyond just the hips will affect their ability to release and move forward. Tight connective tissue from the bottom of the feet, up the back side of the legs, and along the spine to the base of the skull can greatly limit the movement forward.

For these four reasons there is a tendency to injure, pull, or tear the anatomical structures around the hips, causing hip, lower back, and neck pain.

How do I make my forward bends smoother and deeper without tearing or pain?

To create an ease of movement in forward bending so that there is smoothness without hamstring tearing or back pain, follow the eight major principles of movement:

1. Nourish relaxation by breathing and connecting.
2. Initiate movement at the spine.
3. Connect spinal movement with moving through the largest joints first.
4. Move your joints through their optimum range of motion.
5. Create core stability by boosting up your bandhas and breathing.
6. Be relaxed and resilient.
7. Be generous with yourself and move through your pain-free range of motion.
8. Remember that less is more.

In addition to these eight principles of movement, explore the six principles associated specifically with forward bends.

Principles Specific to Forward Bends

1. Relax

Because it is so easy to move into a forward bend quickly and so easy to adjust oneself with a high degree of ambition, it is easy to create injury and dysfunction. So, to be safe, to inspire functional movement and a balanced body, it is important to cultivate awareness of movement.

Breathe and relax before moving into any forward bend. Being relaxed heightens awareness of the bottom of the feet, the inner thighs, the movment of the hip sockets, the movement of the spine, and the amount of leverage the arms are using to pull the body further and deeper. It also allows for inner cues of what is working and what is not working to surface.

2. Initiate Flexion at the Hip Sockets

Forward bends are a recipe for grace and patience. As mentioned earlier, in order to experience a forward bend, the hips must flex. Without hip flexion, the forward bend will not occur.

To optimize forward bending, begin at the hips – literally. Think of sticking out your bum.

A direct application with Uttanasana (Standing Forward Bend)

In order to stick out your bum so that movement is initiated at the hips, simultaneously bend your knees while sticking out your bum; make sure there is no pain or strain in your lower back. The result will have your upper body folded onto your thighs, with your torso resting on your quadriceps and your knees bent. Keeping your torso on the quadriceps, begin to straighten your legs. As the legs straighten, maintain your torso on the quadriceps, allowing for pure movement at the hips. This positioning does a few things anatomically:

- Since you are not moving with gravity in the same way as if you did a swan dive into Uttanasana, it enables you to feel pada bandha and access your core stability (see principle 5).
- It gives you direct experience of the abdominal muscles in forward bends and illustrates how core stability is accessed without "sucking in your abs".
- It prevents any locking of the knees. Locking of the knees can lead to hyperextension. When the knees are in hyperextension the position of the head of the femur in the hip socket can be misaligned, leading to dysfunction in the pelvis and further up the spine.
- It enables pure movement at the hips. The point at which your torso lifts off your thighs is the point at which you can see what is working and what is not working.

3. Balance the External Rotators and Adductors of the Hip

The muscles influencing hip movement include the hip flexors and extensors, hip abductors and adductors, and hip rotators. For optimal movement into a forward bend, there must be balance between them all.

Where to start?

There are two places to start simultaneously – the hip external rotators and the hip adductors. Together, these muscles provide a foundation for a safer and deeper forward bend.

Hip External (Lateral) Rotators
Piriformis, Quadratus Femoris, Obturator Internus and Externus, Gemellus Superior and Inferior

The six external rotators of the hips can be described as fans. They all come together on the femur and fan out around and through the pelvis. They are introduced on page 38 in the discussion on the connection of the hips to the spine, where they are described as muscles that both externally rotate and stabilize the head of the femur in the hip socket. Attaching to both the femur and the pelvis, they connect to the spine by way of the piriformis, which attaches to the sacrum.

As they relate to forward bends, the external rotators of the hips limit hip flexion when they are tight. If they are tight, two things occur:

- The head of the femur rotates externally. This causes the whole thigh to roll outward, away from the midline of the body.
- The pelvis rotates posteriorly. When the pelvis rotates posteriorly, it tucks under – the pubic bone moves toward the navel and the ischial tuberosities move toward the floor.

Let's take a moment to feel it:

Take a moment and move into this pelvic tucked or posteriorly rotated position. Maintaining it, try to forward bend. Feel what happens. Do you move as far into your forward bend?

Hip Adductors
Pectineus, Gracilis, Adductor Brevis, Adductor Longus, Adductor Magnus

The hip adductors were introduced on pages 38 and 41 as muscles associated with pelvic balance as well as with creating core stability through mula bandha. All of the hip adductors originate from the pelvis. Most, except for the gracilis, attach along the femur. The gracilis attaches below the knee on the tibia.

As they relate to forward bends, the hip adductors have a secondary role as medial rotators. Not only do they bring the legs together, they also rotate them inward. As such, when the hip adductors are gently used in forward bends they act as antagonists, balancing the action of the external rotators and helping to create core stability, enabling both the external rotators and the hamstrings to release further.

A direct application with Sukhasana (Simple Seated Cross-Legged Pose) and Dandasana (Staff Pose)

Sitting in Sukhasana (Simple Seated Cross-Legged Pose), tight adductors and tight external rotators create the following posture:

- Knees raised, often higher than the hips (tight adductors)
- Pelvis rotated posteriorly (tight external rotators)

Sitting in Dandasana (Staff Pose), tight external rotators and weak adductors create the following posture:

- Legs rolled outward (tight external rotators and weak adductors)
- Pelvis rotated posteriorly (tight external rotators)

In both of these postures, the spine will also be rounded because the pelvis is not in a neutral position.

Let's add forward flexion and explore what can happen:

With these starting positions, forward flexion at the hips is blocked, so movement forward tends to occur in the spine. Flexion at the spine without flexion at the hips increases the potential to create strain in the spinal discs, SI joint, lower back, and neck.

To regain balance between the external rotators and adductors of the hips, continue reading the next two principles: release connective tissue and engage your core stability.

4. Release Connective Tissue on the Entire Back Side of Your Body

Connective tissue was introduced in section 1 on pages 7–9 and 14–15. As an organizing structure that surrounds, connects, and networks anatomical pieces, its relative tightness will impact movement into a forward bend. Specifically, the connective tissue on the back side of the body includes

- the plantar fascia on the bottom of the feet,
- the fascia surrounding and in the area of the gastrocnemius and soleus muscles,
- the fascia surrounding and in the area of the hamstrings, and
- the thoracolumbar fascia of the back and along the spine to the base of the skull.

When the fascia is tight in these areas, forward bending becomes more limited.

How do I release the fascia on the back side of my body?

Utilizing a simple tool – a tennis ball – will help release the fascia in each of these areas.

1	2	3	4
While standing, roll the tennis ball under the bottom of each foot for two minutes each. This will release the plantar fascia.	While sitting, roll the tennis ball under the back and side of the calf for two minutes on each side. Pay particular attention to the "sweet spots" that make you grimace. Relax your face, and breathe easily. This will release the fascia around the gastrocnemius and around the peroneal muscles.	While sitting, place your right butt cheek on the tennis ball. Roll on the tennis ball with your butt cheek. Again, pay attention to the sweet spots. This will release the fascia around the external rotators and gluteal muscles. Switch to the left side.	While standing against a wall, place the tennis ball between the wall and your back. Roll the ball up and down your back, along your spine and further away from the spine. This will release the thoracolumbar fascia.

Now move into your forward bends. Feel what happens.
Do you go deeper with effortless effort? Do you feel more at ease?

5. Engage Your Core Stability by Activating Pada Bandha and the Hip Adductors

Core stability is important for all yoga asanas, and particularly with forward bends because of the impact of gravity. To control the body's forward movement with gravity, the hamstrings and erector spinae contract eccentrically. As a result, there is less chance for full release. However, if core stability is engaged, release is greater.

There are two key components to creating core stability in forward bends:

• The base of the feet
• The hip adductors

The Feet

The feet are discussed more thoroughly in standing poses. As they relate to forward bends, the positioning of the feet impacts the action of the ankle, which impacts the positioning of the tibia, the knee, and the femur. To activate the feet to create core stability, try the following:

Feel the ball of the foot, the base of the pinky toe, and the center of the heel on both feet. You do not need to press through these points with great strength; just gently bring your awareness to these areas, and the posture of your legs will shift to help solidify your core stability and deepen the forward bend.

The Hip Adductors

The hip adductors are a key group of muscles in core stability. When they are engaged, they have a direct impact on some of the external rotators and the pelvic floor.

6. Leverage Your Arms Only After the Hips Have Moved Their Full Range of Motion

For the arms to assist the forward bend to become deeper, their action must be connected to the movement of the hips as the hips relate to the spine. If it is not connected to the movement of the hips, leveraging the arms causes undue strain on the muscles of the lower and mid-back, of the neck, and along the spine.

A direct application with Uttanasana (Standing Forward Bend)

To move into Uttanasana (Standing Forward Bend) (fig 4-19), the hamstrings and erector spinae control the movement forward by contracting eccentrically. To activate core stability consider the following:

Place two pressed foam blocks or one wooden block between your inner thighs, about one inch from the pelvis. Be sure the blocks are not touching your knees. Gently squeeze the blocks. With the gentle squeeze, the hip adductors are engaged, which co-contracts with mula bandha. The back of the pelvic floor releases, the front of the pelvic floor strengthens and stabilizes, and external rotators release, causing the pelvis to anteriorly rotate and freeing the femur/acetabulum, allowing for the forward bend to move deeper.

Leveraging safely into a forward bend brings in some elements of the back bend.

Let's take a look:

To leverage safely, the movement of the arms and shoulders needs to accentuate the movement of the hips so that forward flexion occurs more deeply between the femur and the acetabulum of the pelvis. To most effectively accomplish this, move the spine and shoulder girdle into a gentle extension by extending at the thoracic spine, then utilize the grasp of the hands/fingers on the toes, feet, and shins to coax more movement between the head of the femur and acetabulum of the pelvis. The idea is to extend the lower back no further than its natural curve, thereby preventing injury along the back side of the body caused by overflexion of the spine.

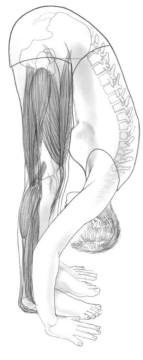

Fig 4-19 Uttanasana (Standing Forward Bend)

twists

Twists are profoundly delightful.

Where back bends are delicious and forward bends are gracious, twists are profoundly delightful. They take us deep into the spine – rotating, twisting, squeezing, strengthening, and releasing all the tissue that lies along the midline of the body. The effects of twists can be felt with even a brief practice – just one or two asanas midday can help release locked-up tension that occurs from daily activities at home or work. Twists indeed feel great. The delightful exclamation in a student's voice as the twist releases tight, tense areas is as if freedom has been born from within. Almost immediately, the upper body stands more upright with greater ease and relief.

The effects of twists can be felt with even a brief practice – just one or two asanas midday can help release locked-up tension that occurs from daily activities at home or work.

This incredibly awesome feeling that twists unleash can also lead to a certain addiction of going deeper. With addiction comes the potential for dysfunction and possible injury. For example, depth in twists before the body is ready can shift the mechanics of the shoulder girdle and pelvic girdle as they relate to the spine. In the shoulder girdle, depth too soon can lead to instability of the scapulae. Instability of the scapulae does not bode well for moving into other asanas such as back bends or inversions. In the pelvic girdle, twisting deeply too soon can lead a student to over-twist the pelvis, creating an imbalance of the SI joint. So it is important to begin by relaxing, breathing, and setting the foundation. Be gentle as you consider the primary action of a twist – rotation of the spine. Then, when you do initiate movement, begin with the spine in mind.

Twists: Rotation of the Spine

In order for a twist to occur, rotation of the spine must occur.

Rotation of the spine involves the action of six muscles. *(fig 4-20 and fig 4-21)* All twists require the following six muscles, whether the twist occurs while seated, standing, supine, or inverted:

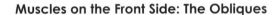

- On the front and side
  - internal obliques
  - external obliques
- On the back
  - rhomboids
  - middle trapezius
  - lower trapezius
- Connecting the front and back
  - serratus anterior

Muscles on the Front Side: The Obliques

The oblique muscles are arranged in layers. The deeper layer consists of the internal obliques, and the superficial layer consists of the external obliques. If you take your fingers and pinch the side of your body between your ribs and the top of the pelvis, you will feel a layer of muscle under the skin and connective tissue. That layer of muscle you are feeling is the external oblique.

What do the obliques look like and how do they work?

Similar to the trapezius muscle, both sets of obliques have groups of fibers that run in distinct directions. So just as we divide the trapezius into the upper, middle, and lower fibers, we can attach similar labels to the fibers of the obliques.

External Obliques: Anterior and Lateral Fibers

The anterior fibers of the external obliques attach to the rib cage from the 5th to 8th ribs, where they interweave with the serratus anterior. They run downward and diagonally toward the linea alba where, through fascia, they also attach.

The lateral fibers of the external obliques attach lower on the rib cage from the 9th to 12th ribs. Running more up and down between the rib cage and pelvis, they also interweave with the serratus anterior. They attach to the front side of the iliac crest, up to the anterior superior iliac spine.

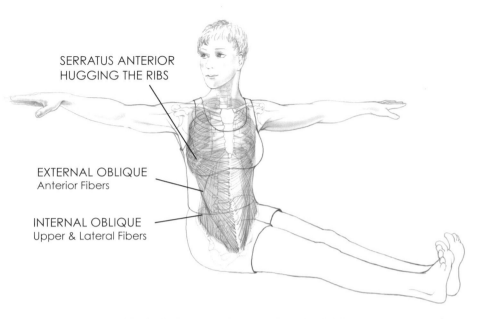

Fig 4-20 The anterior muscles of a twist

Internal Obliques: Lower Anterior, Upper Anterior, and Lateral Fibers

The lower anterior fibers of the internal obliques run parallel to the transversus abdominis.

The upper anterior fibers attach to the pelvis at the iliac crest and fan upward and diagonally toward the linea alba where, through fascia, they attach.

The lateral fibers attach to the iliac crest and the lumbar dorsal fascia at the bottom and span upward to the 10th to 12th ribs.

The Partnership of the Internal and External Obliques to Create a Great Twist

The internal and external obliques have an interesting relationship. When the anterior fibers work together and concentrically contract, forward flexion of the spine is created and the body rounds forward. When the internal and external oblique on one side concentrically contract together, they create a side bend to that same side. When the external oblique on one side and the internal oblique on the other side concentrically contract, they create a twist in the direction of the internal oblique (with the pelvis fixed and stable). For smooth and fluid movement as twists become more complex, gently focus on pure movement between the external oblique on one side and the internal oblique on the other.

Muscles on the Back: The Rhomboids, Middle Trapezius, and Lower Trapezius

The rhomboids and middle trapezius attach on the scapula and the spine *(fig 4-21)*. Arranged in layers, the rhomboids rest deeper to the middle trapezius. Together they help to engage the twist deeper.

Rhomboids

The rhomboids act directly on the scapula. Attaching to the spine from the lower cervical vertebrae and upper thoracic vertebrae and onto the medial border of the scapula, when the rhomboids contract, they pull the scapula toward the spine.

Trapezius – Primarily the Middle Trapezius

The middle trapezius is part of the larger trapezius muscle, which attaches to both the scapula and spine. Specifically, the middle portion of the trapezius lies overtop of the rhomboids, its fibers attaching to the 1st to 5th thoracic vertebrae as well as to the acromion and spine of the scapula. When the middle trapezius contracts it retracts the scapula, bringing it toward the spine.

Muscles Connecting the Front and Back: The Serratus Anterior

The serratus anterior connects the action of the rhomboids and middle trapezius with the action of the obliques to create a fluid, non-ending corkscrew-like motion. Specifically, the serratus anterior attaches to the medial border of the scapula. It links fascially with both the rhomboids and middle trapezius. From the medial border of the scapula, the serratus anterior travels to the lateral side of the body, hugging the rib cage and attaching onto the 1st to 9th ribs. Here it interweaves with the upper portion of the external oblique, making its role as the bridge between the muscles of the back and the front complete *(fig 4-22)*.

The Corkscrew Action of the Twist

Whether the twist is initiated from the top or bottom of the body, the corkscrew action is continuous. For reference let's begin at the bottom and twist right. Assume the pelvis is fixed. Initiating a right twist involves the following actions:

- The right internal oblique contracts.
- The left external oblique contracts.
- The left serratus anterior contracts.
- The left middle trapezius and rhomboids release.
- The right middle trapezius and rhomboids contract.
- The right serratus anterior releases.

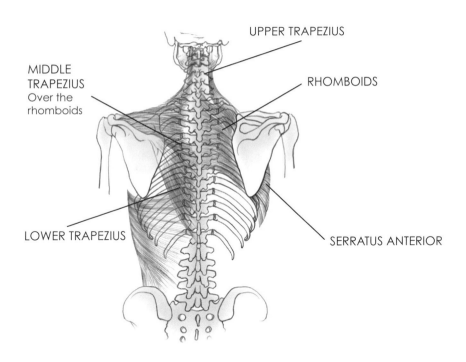

Fig 4-21 The postenor muscles of the twist

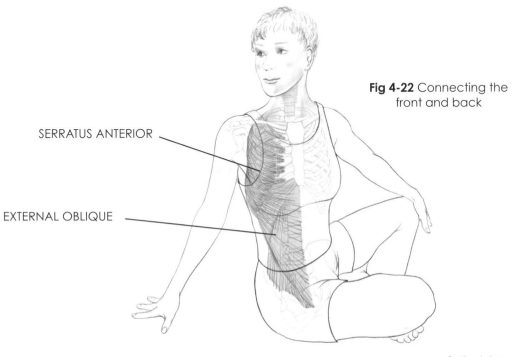

Fig 4-22 Connecting the front and back

Getting Stuck in a Twist

While twists can be simple to move into, they are not always easy. Sometimes, it feels as if the body is stuck, as if it just won't move further. In our minds, we feel we can go further, but physically the rotating action of the spine is not occurring. As a result, we tend to compensate in order to complete the pose – to go deeper, to go further, to twist more. Moving in this way can lead to injuries of the spine, shoulder girdle, pelvic girdle, and rib cage as well as nondescript pain in the back or neck.

Why does this happen?

1

The curves of the spine and the alignment of the vertebrae

The cervical curve rotates more than the thoracic curve, which rotates more than the lumbar curve. This variation is mostly due to the curves of the spine, the size of the vertebrae, and how the vertebral bodies of the vertebrae within each spinal curve interrelate.

The connection between the vertebral bodies of the vertebrae helps transfer weight through the spine. If rotation occurs through the vertebral bodies, there will be more rotation. If it occurs either anterior or posterior to the vertebral bodies, rotation will be limited.

In the cervical curve, most of the rotation occurs between C1 and C2. During development, the vertebral bodies of C1 and C2 fuse together, and C2 acts as a pivot point for rotation of the skull. In the thoracic curve, the alignment of the vertebrae is such that the axis of rotation for twisting passes just perfectly through its vertebral bodies, which allows for a greater ability to rotate. The lumbar spine, on the other hand, has the axis of rotation further back at the base of the spinous processes. This minimizes the amount of rotation available.

2

Overuse of the neck in twists

Since the cervical spine is the easiest place to move in a twist, two things tend to happen:

• It often becomes the primary source of movement when the torso is stiff or stuck. This can restrict the opportunity to fully release and strengthen the rest of the torso, creating imbalance between the cervical, thoracic, and lumbar spines.

• It becomes more difficult to wait. Where the eyes gaze, the body wants to go. If the body is stiff or stuck and unable to follow the gaze of the eyes, compensation by over-leveraging with the arms or over-rotating at the cervical spine can lead to injury in the neck and shoulder girdle.

3

General posture

As with back bends, the posture of kyphosis, or forward rounding of the spine, limits twisting. This is due to two reasons:

• Kyphosis changes the relationship between each of the thoracic vertebrae, so the axis of rotation changes.

• Kyphosis can create weakness and tightness of the muscles associated with twisting, causing imbalances. As the muscles become less balanced, rotating tends to become more limited.

For these three reasons, there is a tendency to compensate by over-leveraging the arms, overcontracting muscles of the neck, destabilizing the structures of the shoulder girdle, and over-rotating through the pelvis, all of which can cause tension and dysfunction in the neck, back, and shoulders.

How do I make my twists smoother, deeper, and easier?

To ensure smooth and easy movement of your twists, follow the eight major principles of movement:

1. Nourish relaxation by breathing and connecting.
2. Initiate movement at the spine.
3. Connect spinal movement with moving through the largest joints first.
4. Move your joints through their optimum range of motion.
5. Create core stability by boosting up your bandhas and breathing.
6. Be relaxed and resilient.
7. Be generous with yourself and move through your pain-free range of motion.
8. Remember that less is more.

In addition to these eight principles of movement, explore the five principles associated specifically with twists.

Principles Specific to Twisting

1. Relax

Relaxing and breathing before moving into any twist brings awareness to your base of support, your foundation from which the twist emerges. A twist primarily occurs in the spine, so whatever your base – your feet, legs, pelvis, arms, or hands – it needs to be solid.

Applying anatomy to asanas: To create a solid base, bring awareness to it and imagine its energetic roots sinking into the floor and into the earth; then feel the earth's energy coming back into you. This will help connect you to your base, allowing your spine to more freely rotate.

Once in movement, breathing will help continue the movement. The diaphragm is fascially connected to the serratus anterior. The serratus anterior is connected to the external oblique.

If the diaphragm is easily moving, chances are better that the serratus anterior and external oblique will also move with greater ease.

2. Initiate Movement from Your Core: Move Your Neck Last

Twists, like back bends, provide a sumptuous space for exploring the spine. As mentioned earlier, rotation occurs through the spine. Without it, a twist will be difficult to experience. So, when moving into your twist, begin by moving at the abdomen, then sequentially up the torso, and then into the neck. By moving in this way, mobility and strength can be sequentially developed, improving posture and body balance, all while preventing injury.

Why begin at the abdomen?

Initiating rotation at the abdomen causes the following to happen:

1	2
It allows the rib cage to connect with the top of the pelvis, rather than being slouched so the ribs point inward toward the belly or extended so the ribs flare out. With the ribs connected to the pelvis, the obliques are in a prime position for rotating.	The transversus abdominis, which provides support to the spine, is more readily engaged as compared to when the body is slouched forward or overly extended with the ribs flared out. This helps prevent spinal collapse.

Applying anatomy to asanas: Whether you are sitting, standing, or inverted, bring awareness to your navel area. Feel its connection as a lotus flower, with petals expanding open, downward toward the pubic bone, hip sockets, anterior superior iliac spine, and sacrum. Next imagine the petals expanding outward to the lateral edges of your torso, upward toward either side of your rib cage, and directly upward toward the sternum. Allow this lotus flower to remain bloomed open as you initiate and continue the twist. You will feel the subtle lift that emerges from this image.

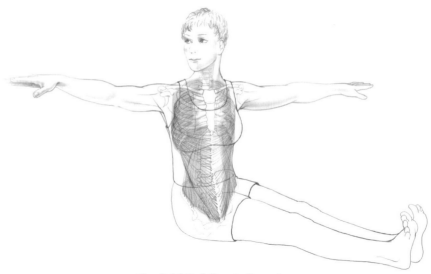

Fig 4-23 Twisting in Dandasana
with arms at shoulder height

A direct application with a twist

A simple seated twist best explores this concept, and once it is mastered, it can be used in all twists.

Begin in a seated position *(fig 4-23)*. You can be in a simple cross-legged position or with your legs out as in Dandasana (Staff Pose). Take your arms to shoulder height, or place your hands on your shoulders or on your head. Feel your breath and experience your spine. If you feel yourself slouching, sit up on a block. If you feel that you are sitting tall with effortless effort, then you are ready. Allow your lotus flower to bloom in your abdomen.

- As you exhale, begin to twist right, from your navel and solar plexus. Your obliques will be activated.
- Initially, keep your nose in line with your navel.
- Be sure you are still sitting on your ischial tuberosities.
- Allow your chest to stay open. Ideally, the lotus flower of your abdomen will support your chest to be open. This allows your postural muscles to support you while you twist.
- Relax your shoulders, relaxing the muscles of your neck.
- Be sure your knees are still in the same place. Ensure that one knee hasn't moved further forward.
- Now, begin to retract the right shoulder blade. Your middle trapezius and rhomboids will contract. Let the left shoulder blade protract. The left middle trapezius and rhomboids will release, and the left serratus anterior will contract. Be sure you are doing this with ease, with little tension.
- Be sure that your shoulders are not elevating toward your ears. If they are, then you are compensating.
- Release. Switch sides.

3. After the Abdomen Moves, Lead with the Chest, Then Connect the Arm and Neck Movement with the Spine

Once movement has been initiated in the twist, continue by leading with the chest before bringing in the arms or neck. Sometimes this is difficult because the thoracic spine is tight. If the muscles of the chest are tight or desensitized, or if there is a tendency for the scapulae to ride up to the ears and the shoulders to round forward, it may be difficult to lead with the chest.

Benefits of Leading with the Chest and Then Adding the Arms and Neck

There are several benefits of leading with the chest before initiating movement of the arms and neck:

- Continues to strengthen the obliques, rhomboids, middle trapezius, serratus anterior
- Can release the stuck areas of the thoracic spine
- Ensures the neck doesn't over-rotate
- Ensures the arms don't over-leverage, creating strain through the torso

A direct application with Marichyasana (Pose Dedicated to the Sage Marichi)

Let's move into Marichyasana (Pose Dedicated to the Sage Marichi) *(fig 4-24)*. To move fully into Marichyasana, the spine needs to rotate the torso around about 90 degrees. The arms help to leverage the pose deeper. If the arms leverage before the shoulder girdle or spine is ready, injury can occur. Let's take a look:

In creating depth in twists, spinal rotation and shoulder girdle stability are connected. The spine needs to rotate sufficiently, and the humerus needs to connect with the movement of the scapula. If the rotation of the spine is not sufficient, the humerus needs to reach further to grasp the knee. In Marichyasana, this can lead to a tendency to elevate the scapula and roll the shoulder forward. When that happens, a slouch occurs and strain or injury can ensue.

Try this: Sit with your left knee up and your right leg straight. Use a block if you need to support your pelvis or if your hips are tight. Establish your foundation. On the exhale, initiate from your abdomen and twist toward your bent knee. This will engage your obliques. From the obliques, allow the chest to move. This will engage the rhomboids, middle trapezius, and serratus anterior. If you are sufficiently rotated, place your elbow on the outside of the knee – without elevating your shoulder blade or rolling your shoulder forward. Maintain the connection between the arm and the scapula as you gently press the arm against the knee/leg and the knee/leg against the arm. Keep the shoulder girdle relaxed.

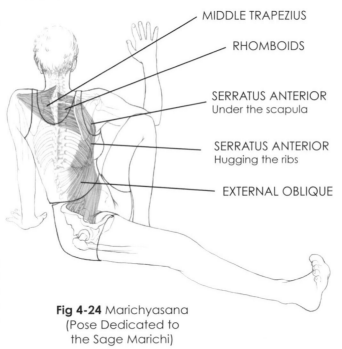

MIDDLE TRAPEZIUS

RHOMBOIDS

SERRATUS ANTERIOR
Under the scapula

SERRATUS ANTERIOR
Hugging the ribs

EXTERNAL OBLIQUE

Fig 4-24 Marichyasana (Pose Dedicated to the Sage Marichi)

4. Stabilize the Connection between the Pelvis and the Spine

Sometimes it is difficult to initiate from the abdomen and continue with the chest when in standing twists because the muscles of the lower back are tight or desensitized, the pelvis is unstable, or the hips are tight. When the lower back is dysfunctional, there is a tendency for the pelvis to move with dysfunction as well. Whichever the situation, there is a greater

chance for injury. By improving the connection between the pelvis and spine and between the pelvis and femurs, you can gain a foundational structure from which your twist can move safely and easily.

How do I do this?

Follow these steps to stabilize the pelvis:

1

Balance the rotation action of the obliques, serratus anterior, rhomboids, and middle trapezius with the support of the transversus abdominis, multifidi, hip adductors, and anterior pelvic floor muscles.

2

Connect the action of the hamstrings, gluteus maximus, and lumbar spine with the balance of the hip rotators.

A direct application with Trikonasana (Triangle Pose)

Let's explore this with Trikonasana (Triangle Pose) from Parsvottanasana (Pyramid Pose), with the left leg forward and the right leg back. Specific to Trikonasana and all twists that have the legs straight (whether sitting, standing, or inverted), a stable pelvis will create a solid twist.

In this pose, the difficulty lies in the foundation, in maintaining the base of support. When the base of support is a combination of the feet, legs, and pelvis, as in a standing twist, it becomes easier to over-rotate and overcompensate through the pelvis and SI joint rather than move through the obliques, serratus anterior, middle trapezius, and rhomboids. When that occurs, there is a greater possibility for back pain.

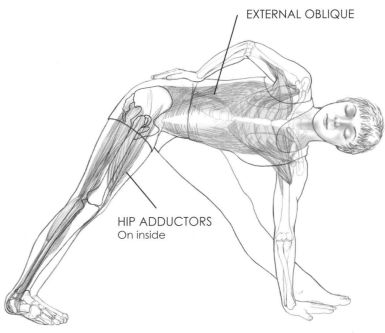

EXTERNAL OBLIQUE

HIP ADDUCTORS
On inside

Fig 4-25 Trikonasana
(Triangle Pose)

Let's take a look:

Pelvic Stability: Transversus Abdominis, Obliques, Multifidi, Hip Adductors, Anterior Pelvic Floor

With the legs in Trikonasana (Triangle Pose) *(fig 4-25)*, imagine the upper thighs like scissors. The heads of the fémurs are moving together, like the top portion of scissors. Or, you can place a rolled mat between your upper thighs. The resulting action from either of these ideas will help to gently contract the anterior portion of the pelvic floor, transversus abdominis, internal obliques, and multifidi, along with the hip adductors *(external oblique and hip adductors shown in fig 4-25)*. If any of these muscles are weak, if the contraction is unbalanced, or if the muscles are contracted with too much force and without breath, the foundational stability of the pelvis will be compromised, leading to poor pelvic stability, dysfunctional movement, possible pain, and potential injury.

Continuing the Twist from a Stable Pelvis: Connecting the Pelvis with the Rotation of the Spine

From the foundation, with the left leg forward, place your left hand on the inside of your left thigh. Be sure your spine is in neutral. Place your right hand on the back of your sacrum. This will ensure your pelvis stays in neutral.

Now, start to twist beginning at the abdomen. Then gently swivel the chest. If you feel your lower back arch, ease out. This means you are moving into extension rather than rotating.

At this point you will be in Trikonasana, your spine rotated with your nose in line with your navel. To explore moving your neck in order to rotate your head upward, read on....

5. Adding the Neck: Connect It with the Movement of the Chest and Abdomen

Adding the neck is intuitive for the body when the abdomen and chest are in the correct position and the pelvis is balanced. Adding the neck begins by connecting the rhomboids with muscles of the neck that cause rotation. There are many, including splenius capitis and cervicis, longissimus capitis and cervicis, longus capitis, longus colli, rectus capitis anterior, sternocleidomastoid, scalenes, and upper trapezius. Many of these muscles also allow for extension or flexion of the cervical spine as well, so when rotating, allow your attention to nurture pure rotation.

The smooth action of the neck is influenced by the action and stability of the shoulder girdle (more on this in inversions). So as you move from the abdomen to the chest to the neck in twists, be sure to remain stable in the chest for easy movement of the neck.

A direct application with Trikonasana (Triangle Pose)

From Trikonasana (Triangle Pose), be sure your pelvis remains stable. The previous exploration ended with the left leg in flexion, the right leg in extension, the left hand on the inside of the left thigh, and the right hand on the back of the sacrum. From an open chest, gently raise your right arm to the ceiling, while keeping the humerus connected to the movement of the scapula. Spiral your chest to the ceiling. Notice if both sides of your chest – front and back; left and right – feel equally open. That is what you want. If you feel equally open, then rotate your neck to enable your eyes to look at your fingers. Switch sides. Notice how you feel.

Breathing Out -
  Touching the Root of Heaven,
One's heart opens;
  The Dragon slips into the water.
Breathing In -
  Standing on the Root of Earth,
One's heart is still and deep;
  The Tiger's claw cannot be moved.

— *Source unknown*

inversions

Inversions create lightness.

Inversions take us into an arena that is separate from back bends, forward bends, and twists. They shake us up by shifting perspective, posture, and muscular coordination. By doing so, they create lightness.

As humans, we maintain an upright position for most of our day, either standing, sitting, or walking, with a mostly forward-facing perspective, feet on the ground. The lower limbs hold the body's weight, and the eyes take in the world that rests in front and to the periphery – this includes the world that exists when looking up, down, or to the side.

Inversions take us into an arena that is separate from back bends, forward bends, and twists. They shake us up by shifting perspective, posture, and muscular coordination. By doing so, they create lightness.

Being upside down shifts that. In an inverted position, the arms and hands work like the legs and feet. Their role changes from one of gesture to one of weight-bearing. The shoulder girdle functions as the pelvic girdle, transferring the weight of the body through to the arms and hands. The head becomes limited in its range of motion, so rather than following visual distractions, the line of sight becomes gently focused. This shift in function can create incredible upper body strength. However, if the connection between the shoulder girdle and the spine is dysfunctional, it can lead to compression of the cervical vertebrae and repetitive strain issues in the elbows and wrists.

Inversions: The Spine, Shoulder Girdle, and Arms

All inversions share three commonalities:

- The spine is upside down.
- The arms bear the body's weight.
- The shoulder girdle, arms, and hands provide the foundation from which the inversion occurs.

Developing a Foundation

Inversions can balance on the upper arms, shoulders, and upper back as in Salamba Sarvangasana (Shoulder Stand) (fig 4-26); on the head or the head and forearms as in Sirsasana (Headstand) (fig 4-27); or on just the forearms as in Pincha Mayurasana (Forearm Stand) (fig 4-28). While the positioning of the limbs is slightly different in each of these situations, each creates a foundation that strongly connects the shoulder girdle to the arms and the shoulder girdle to the rib cage.

Let's take a look:

Creating Stability in the Shoulder Girdle

We initially explored the shoulder girdle in principle 3, connect spinal movement with movement at the largest joints first, on page 32. There, the shoulder girdle is described as a skeletal structure consisting of the clavicles and scapulae, which are designed and positioned to maximally help the arms move in all directions. When we are inverted, the functioning of the shoulder girdle and its surrounding muscles contributes to strength and stability.

Stability comes from a series of muscles on the front, back, and sides of the body:

- The rhomboids
- The trapezius
- The serratus anterior
- The pectoralis minor
- The levator scapulae
- The latissimus dorsi

Together, the balance of these six muscles keeps the shoulder girdle stable while other muscles move the body into the inverted position. We have discussed these muscles in other sections. For a review of how they work together, you can refer to page 34.

Strong Arms: Connecting the Hands and Arms with the Torso

From this base of stability radiates strength that flows down the arms and into the hands, then rebounds and returns back to the core. Since the positioning of the limbs is slightly different in each inversion, let's take a closer look at each asana and explore the muscles involved in setting up each of their foundational positions.

Salamba Sarvangasana (Shoulder Stand)

No matter if you enter into Salamba Sarvangasana (fig 4-26) from Setu Bandha Sarvangasana (Little Bridge Pose) or Halasana (Plow Pose), the essence of this asana is a back bend, with the thoracic spine and upper arms moving into extension and the forearms moving in flexion.

Thoracic spine extension occurs when the primary extensors of the thoracic spine contract. The primary extensors are the erector spinae. The lower trapezius also contracts to support the extension by gently pulling the scapulae toward the pelvis.

Upper arm extension is created by a contraction of the extensors of the upper arms, including the latissimus dorsi and teres major, the posterior deltoid, and the long head of the triceps brachii.

Forearm flexion is created from a contraction of the biceps brachii, the brachioradialis, and the brachialis muscles.

To complete each of these movements, other muscles also need to release. Most of these muscles were introduced on pages 33–35 as muscles that connect the arm to the torso. As they release, they help to enable extension of the thoracic spine and extension of the upper arm:

Deep:
- transversus thoracis
- pectoralis minor
- subclavius
- coracobrachialis
- biceps brachii

Superficial:
- pectoralis major

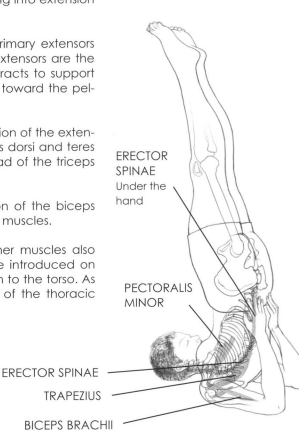

Fig 4-26 Salamba Sarvangasana (Shoulder Stand)

ERECTOR SPINAE
Under the hand

PECTORALIS MINOR

ERECTOR SPINAE

TRAPEZIUS

BICEPS BRACHII

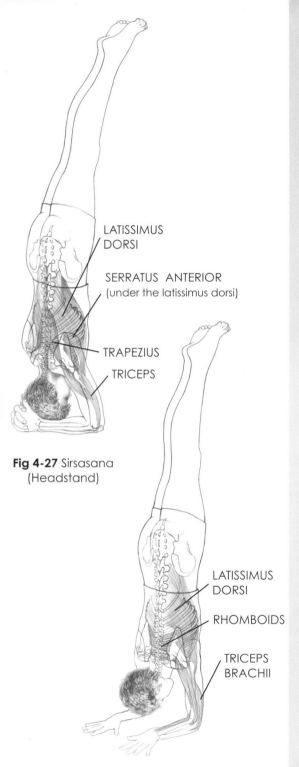

LATISSIMUS DORSI

SERRATUS ANTERIOR
(under the latissimus dorsi)

TRAPEZIUS

TRICEPS

Fig 4-27 Sirsasana (Headstand)

LATISSIMUS DORSI

RHOMBOIDS

TRICEPS BRACHII

Fig 4-28 Pincha Mayurasana (Forearm Stand)

Sirsasana (Headstand)

Where shoulder stands are about strength, headstands *(fig 4-27)* are about balance. Depending on your teacher and style of yoga, head and hand placement will be different. However, no matter how the head or hands are placed, the initial foundation is created by bringing the arms overhead and creating stability through the shoulder girdle, arms, and hands. This occurs through the following:

- Upward rotation of the scapulae
- Flexion of the arms at the shoulder
- Flexion of the forearms at the shoulder
- Internal rotation of the humerus at the shoulder

Upward rotation of the scapula is created by the contraction of the upper fibers of the serratus anterior. With full upward rotation of the scapula, the glenoid fossa points upward, enabling the arm muscles to function more smoothly.

Arm flexion is created by the contraction of the anterior deltoid, biceps brachii, and pectoralis major muscles.

Forearm flexion occurs from a contraction of the biceps brachii, the brachioradialis, and the brachialis muscles.

To enable upward rotation of the scapula, arm flexion, and forearm flexion, the following muscles need to release:

- Rhomboids to enable upward rotation
- Posterior deltoid, triceps, teres major, and some fibers of the latissimus dorsi to enable arm flexion
- Triceps to enable forearm flexion

Once the arms are overhead, they still need to internally rotate at the shoulder in order for the hands to come together. To do this, some of the fibers of the latissimus dorsi and the teres major contract along with the pectoralis major and subscapularis. This contraction is balanced by the release of the external rotators of the shoulders – the infraspinatus and teres minor. It is important to note that while the external rotators need to release in order to initially set up the foundation of the headstand, they will contract to help prevent collapse of the shoulder girdle while in this pose (read more on this in the principles specific to inversions).

Pincha Mayurasana (Forearm Stand)

Pincha Mayurasana (Forearm Stand) *(fig 4-28)* has a similar arm position to Sirsasana (Headstand), without the head as a point of support.

In addition to upward rotation of the scapulae, arm flexion, and forearm flexion, the forearms are also pronated. Pronation is created primarily by the pronator quadratus and the pronator teres. The pronator quadratus is located close to the wrist about one quarter of the way up the arm. You can't actually palpate the muscle; however, if you place two fingers of your left hand on the palmar side of your right wrist as if you are taking your pulse, you would be over top of the pronator quadratus. The pronator teres lies just below the elbow. More superficial than the pronator quadratus, this muscle can be palpated by placing your left thumb about two finger widths below your right elbow joint on the palmar side. Press firmly and slowly pronate your arm, turning the palm of your hand to the floor. What you feel contracting under your thumb is the pronator teres.

Neck Pain and Wrist Strain: A Result of Weakness and Tightness

No matter which inversion you are moving into, the same primary caution needs to be addressed – slumping through the shoulder girdle, causing pain in the cervical spine or pain and weakness in the elbows and wrists.

Why does this happen?

As with all of the potential problems that can occur with asanas, the tendency toward injury is an honest one. If the appropriate body part doesn't move to bring us into the asana, we subconsciously find another way. This is the path of least resistance, and with inversions it occurs when there is tightness or weakness of the muscles supporting the shoulder girdle.

How does it occur?

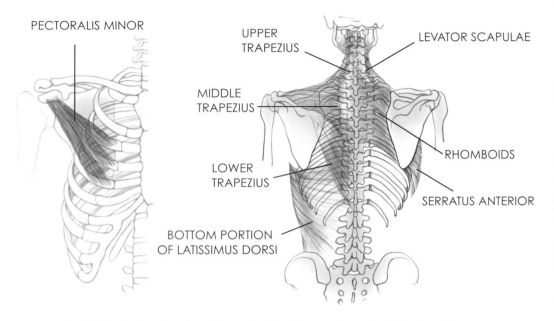

PECTORALIS MINOR

UPPER TRAPEZIUS

LEVATOR SCAPULAE

MIDDLE TRAPEZIUS

LOWER TRAPEZIUS

RHOMBOIDS

SERRATUS ANTERIOR

BOTTOM PORTION OF LATISSIMUS DORSI

Fig 4-29 Muscles involved in protecting the neck and wrist in inversions

1

Imbalance between the serratus anterior, upper trapezius, rhomboids, and levator scapulae (fig 4-29)

Typically, when the serratus anterior and some fibers of the upper trapezius contract and the rhomboids and levator scapulae release, the scapula moves in upward rotation. As they relate to inversions with the arms overhead in Sirsasana (Headstand) and Pincha Mayurasana (Forearm Stand), these four muscles help rotate the scapula upward so that the glenoid fossa of the scapula is pointing almost overhead. Without this scapular rotation, it is impossible to bring the arms overhead. If these muscles are imbalanced, it will be more difficult to maintain the scapular position and, in turn, the foundation of the inversion.

2

Weakness of the external rotators of the shoulder

The external rotators of the shoulder are the infraspinatus and the teres minor, also known as the posterior rotator cuff. When they are tight they contribute to the arm rolling medially. If they are tight or weak when practicing inversions such as Pincha Mayurasana (Forearm Stand), the tightness will cause the elbows to flare out and the hands to slide together. In Sirsasana (Headstand), the hand position will collapse inward, and more weight will land on the head. In Salamba Sarvangasana (Shoulder Stand), the upper arms roll inward, the elbows slide outward, and the pose collapses onto the upper back and neck.

3

Upside down, our perspective is different

One of the easiest ways to find balance in inversions is to move through the three weak links of the spine. That is why you see the common "banana position" in Sirsasana (Headstand) and Pincha Mayurasana (Forearm Stand). It is the easiest way to balance. Unfortunately, as in back bends, continuing to move this way in inversions will actually create more problems in your body.

4

General posture

If there is a tendency toward kyphosis, or a rounded forward position, there is a tendency toward tightening, weakening, and dysfunctional movement patterns. Hunched shoulders and a rounded thoracic spine can create weakness or tightness in the neck muscles and the muscles of the shoulder girdle. This can lead to a less than optimal position of the humerus in the shoulder socket, which can contribute to poor mechanics of the shoulder girdle and a poor foundation for inversions.

For these four reasons, there is a tendency to slump rather than strengthen, leading to potential injury in the wrist, elbows, shoulders, and neck.

How do I stabilize my shoulder girdle to protect my cervical spine and wrists?

For a safely inverted asana that is strong, balanced, and light, follow the eight major principles of movement:

1. Nourish relaxation by breathing and connecting.
2. Initiate movement at the spine.
3. Connect spinal movement with moving through the largest joints first.
4. Move your joints through their optimum range of motion.
5. Create core stability by boosting up your bandhas and breathing.
6. Be relaxed and resilient.
7. Be generous with yourself and move through your pain-free range of motion.
8. Remember that less is more.

In addition to these eight principles of movement, explore the four principles associated specifically with inversions.

Principles Specific to Inversions

1. Relax

Breathe and relax before moving into any inversion. Breathing and relaxing enable you to connect your foundation of hands, arms, shoulder girdle, and/or head to the floor. By connecting you can access the energy rebounding from the floor back into you, which helps move your body up into the pose. It also gives you a moment to gauge where you need to be so that you can transform any apprehension you may have about going upside down.

2. Gently Extend at the Thoracic Spine

Inversions can be scary. They can also add an exhilaration that subtly emerges in the skin and through the body once the asana has come to completion, when the feet are on the floor and the head has slowly come back up. This feeling, due in part to being upside down, can be accentuated by the actions of the spine.

We initially examined and explored the thoracic spine in the section on back bends. In back bends, the recommendation was to initiate movement from the thoracic spine. In inversions, gentle extension at the thoracic spine helps prevent slumping. It leads to your core being engaged and your legs being strongly active to help keep you up and balanced in the inversion.

A direct application with Salamba Sarvangasana (Shoulder Stand)

Salamba Sarvangasana (Shoulder Stand) is perhaps the most obvious of the inversions. Accessed from Setu Bandha Sarvangasana (Little Bridge Pose) or Halasana (Plow Pose), the essence is to balance primarily on the shoulders and upper arms while extending through the thoracic spine.

Opinions vary as to where the pressure is placed on the upper part of the body. Some teachers say it is on the neck, others say on C7 and across to the shoulders and upper arms. For the sake of shoulder stability and safety of the neck, and ease of extension through the thoracic spine, I tend toward balance occurring on the shoulders and upper arms. This enables C7–T1 and the subsequent thoracic vertebrae to easily move into extension.

No matter how you move into Salamba Sarvangasana (Shoulder Stand), the following needs to occur to enable extension through the thoracic spine:

- External rotation of the humerus at the scapula
- Extension of the humerus at the scapula
- Extension of the thoracic spine

To enable external rotation and extension of the humerus and extension of the thoracic spine the following actions must occur:

- Pectoralis minor, coracobrachialis, and biceps brachii release
- Infraspinatus and teres minor contract
- Erector spinae contracts, with support of the lower trapezius

Applying anatomy to asanas: Salamba Sarvangasana (Shoulder Stand) – Consider the principles of back bends, of feeling the breath in the sternum. Not willfully, but gently, as if feeling the lungs rise and fall, causing the rib cage to rise and fall. From that feeling, press both the outside and inside of your upper arms toward the floor. Allow the thoracic spine to soften into your body, and let your lower back settle into your hands. Feel the weight of your body settle along your shoulders toward your elbows. Continue to feel both the outside and inside of your arms gently pressing into the floor.

3. Connect Arm Movement with Shoulder Girdle Movement

Besides fear, one of the difficulties of moving into inversions is the ability to balance on the arms. One factor needed for balance is mobility of the arms in the shoulder joint.

To bring the arms overhead, the humerus moves into flexion at the shoulder joint. To do this, two things occur:

1. The arms must move into flexion.
2. The scapulae must rotate upward.

If one of these two actions does not occur, the arms will not move overhead.

Let's take a look:

To rotate the scapula upward, the serratus anterior and upper trapezius contract while the rhomboids and levator scapulae need to release. To move the arm into flexion, the anterior deltoid, pectoralis major, biceps brachii, and coracobrachialis contract while the posterior deltoid, teres major, and latissimus dorsi release.

To feel this for yourself grab hold of a pressed foam block. Hold it between your forearms so your arms are about shoulder-width apart, with your elbows bent at 90 degrees and in line with your wrists, which are in line with your shoulders. Don't let your elbows slip out to the sides. Maintaining this position, raise the block over your head. Is there any strain with lifting the block over your head?

This movement is similar to the movement in Sirsasana (Headstand) and Pincha Mayurasana (Forearm Stand). If there is strain or if you are compensating for your movement by leaning backward, wiggling, or wobbling, it is possible that there is tightness or weakness in the muscles of your shoulder girdle, which could cause imbalance or dysfunction of your shoulder girdle when in inversions.

4. Optimize Wrist Support – Connect Hand Movement with Shoulder Girdle Stability

Hasta bandha is considered to be the energy lock located in the palm of the hands. It allows the energy to smoothly move from the shoulder girdle to the hands and rebound back toward the shoulder girdle, bringing ease, balance, and strength to the inversion.

Hand movements are precise, delicate, and strong. Their actions are well connected to the movements of the forearm, shoulder girdle, and rib cage. To experience this, lift your hands in front of yourself and supinate and pronate your forearms. Notice how your hands move with your forearms as they roll toward the floor and toward the ceiling. Now externally and internally rotate your humerus at the shoulder girdle. Notice the hand movement. Since the hand is well connected to the shoulder girdle and forearm, our focus will be on exploring these as a means to access the hands.

A direct application with Sirsasana (Headstand)

In creating a safe foundation for headstands, connect with the ulnar ridge of your forearms. To feel this, take your left hand and press into the pinky finger side of your right forearm (fig 4-30). You will feel the ridge of the ulna, or the ulnar ridge, under your fingers. As you move toward your wrist, you will feel the styloid process of the ulna. It is the piece that sticks out slightly at the wrist, on the pinky finger side.

As you set up for a headstand, feel the ulnar ridge and styloid process of your forearms on the floor. This connection puts the forearm halfway between supination and pronation and balances the action of medial and lateral rotation of the humerus. This prevents collapse, which occurs with excessive pronation and medial rotation, as well as prevents tightness, which occurs with excessive supination and lateral rotation.

A direct application with Pincha Mayurasana (Forearm Stand)

This time as you set yourself up, pronate your forearms so that the palmar side of the forearm and hand is in contact with the floor (fig 4-31). Your elbows will be directly in line with your wrists; your shoulders will be above your elbows. As preparation continues and kick-up is imminent, the elbows tend to swing outward. To prevent this, gently activate your external rotators, the teres minor and infraspinatus (be sure to relax your jaw as you do this). This will help ground your forearms into position as you kick up.

Applying anatomy to asanas: Feel the ridge on the pinky side of your forearm and the "sticky outy" on the pinky side of your wrist. Once your fingers are interlaced, connect those two points to the floor. Be sure you are not rolling inward or too far outward. The thumb side of the wrist will be facing toward the ceiling. Stay in contact with this position throughout the movement to ensure that your arms are not rolling in or out. As your arms become tired, you may feel a slight inward or outward roll. That is a strong cue to come out of the pose.

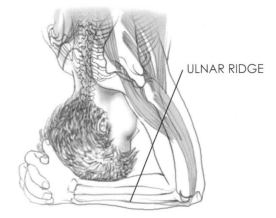

ULNAR RIDGE

Fig 4-30 Connect with the ulnar ridge

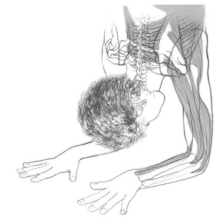

Fig 4-31 Contact floor with palms

There is one way of breathing

that is shameful and constricted.

Then there's another way;

a breath of love that takes you

all the way to infinity.

— *Rumi*

Notes:

Section 1

   1. Martini, F., M. Timmons, and M. McKinley. 2000. *Human Anatomy*. 3rd edition. New Jersey: Prentice Hall. p. 64.
   2. Ibid., p. 74.
   3. Ibid., p. 212-213.
   4. Biel, A. 1997. *Trail Guide to the Body*. Self-Published.

Section 2

   1. Janda, Vladimir. 1983. *Muscle Function Testing*. Butterworths.

Section 3

   1. Johnson, W. 2000. *Aligned, Relaxed, Resilient*. Boston: Shambala.
   2. First heard in a conversation with Lorrie Maffey, PT.
   3. Taught to me by Dr. Karandikar, Yoga Instructor.
   4. Myers, T. 2001. *Anatomy Trains*. London: Churchill Livingstone. p. 159-181.
   5. Ibid.
   6. Moore, Kevin L. 1992. *Clinically Oriented Anatomy*. 3rd edition. Baltimore: Williams & Wilkins. p. 250.
   7. This concept developed out of a conversation with Lorrie Maffey, PT.
   8. Swami Buddhananda. 1998. *Moola Bandha*. Varanasi, UP, India: Bhargava Bhushan Press. p. 80-84.
   9. Taught to me first by Swati Fernandez.
 10. Taught to me first by Margot Kitchen in her Pranayama workshops.
 11. Martini, F., and E. Bartholomew. 2000. *Essentials of Anatomy and Physiology*. 2nd edition. New Jersey: Prentice Hall. p. 180.

Section 4

   1. First heard in a workshop with Margot Kitchen.

bibliography

Barral, Jean Pierre. 1991. *The Thorax*.
Seattle: Eastland Press.

Biel, A. 1997. *Trail Guide to the Body*.
Self-Published.

Caillet, Rene. 1985. *Knee Pain and Disability*.
Philadelphia: F.A. Davis.

Calais-Germain, B. 1993. *Anatomy of Movement*.
Seattle: Eastland Press.

Coulter, David H. 2001. *Anatomy of Hatha Yoga*.
Honesdale, PA: Body and Breath.

Dimon, Theodore, Jr. 2001. *Anatomy of the Moving Body*. Berkeley, CA: North Atlantic Books.

Dossey, Larry. 1982. Space, *Time and Medicine*. Boston: New Science Library.

Downie, Patricia, ed. 1986. *Cash's Textbook of Neurology for Physiotherapists*. 4th edition.
Great Britain: Faber & Faber.

Fahri, D. 1996. *The Breathing Book*.
New York: Henry Holt.

Fahri, D. 2000. *Yoga Mind, Body & Spirit*.
New York: Henry Holt.

Feldenkrais, M. 1977. *Awareness through Movement*. New York: Penguin Books.

Feldenkrais, M. 1977. *The Case of Nora*.
New York: Harper & Row.

Frawley, David. 2001. *Secrets of the 5 Pranas*.
Santa Fe, NM: American Institute of Vedic Studies.

Holleman, Dona, and O. Sen-Gupta. 1999.
Dancing the Body of Light.
The Netherlands: Pegasus Enterprises.

Iyengar, B.K.S. 1979. *Light on Yoga*.
New York: Schocken Books.

Janda, Vladimir. 1983. *Muscle Function Testing*. Butterworths.

Johnson, W. 2000. *Aligned, Relaxed, Resilient*.
Boston: Shambala.

Juhan, D. 1987. *Job's Body*. Barrytown,
NY: Station Hill Press.

Kendall, F., E. McCreary, and P. Provance. 1993.
Muscles, Testing and Function. 4th edition.
Baltimore: Williams & Wilkins.

Krastof, Gary. 1999. *Yoga for Wellness*.
New York: Penguin Group.

Lasater, Judith. 1995. *Relax and Renew*.
Berkeley, CA: Rodmell Press.

Martini, F., and E. Bartholomew. 2000. *Essentials of Anatomy and Physiology*. 2nd edition.
New Jersey: Prentice Hall.

Martini, F., M. Timmons, and M. McKinley. 2000.
Human Anatomy. 3rd edition.
New Jersey: Prentice Hall.

Moore, Kevin L. 1992. *Clinically Oriented Anatomy*. 3rd edition. Baltimore: Williams & Wilkins.

Moyers, B. 1993. *Healing and the Mind*.
New York: Doubleday.

Myers, T. 1997–2000. *Body Cubed*. A collection of bound magazine articles published in Massage Magazine.

Myers, T. 2001. *Anatomy Trains*.
London: Churchill Livingstone.

Perry, J., D. Rohe, and A. Garcia. 1996.
The Kinesiology Workbook. 2nd edition.
Philadelphia: F.A. Davis.

Rasch, P., and R. Burke. 1976. *Kinesiology and Applied Anatomy*. 5th edition.
Philadelphia: Lea & Febiger.

Robin, Mel. 2002. *A Physiological Handbook for Teachers of Yogasana*.
Tucson, AZ: Fenestra Books.

Schiffmann, E. 1996. *Yoga*.
New York: Simon & Schuster.

Schultz, L., and R. Feitis. 1996. *The Endless Web*.
Berkeley, CA: North Atlantic Books.

Smith, L., E. Weiss, and L.D. Lehmkuhl. 1996.
Brunnstrom's Clinical Kinesiology. 5th edition.
Philadelphia: F.A. Davis.

Spence, Alexander. 1990. *Basic Human Anatomy*. 3rd edition.
Redwood City, CA: Benjamin Cummings Publishing.

Stark, Steven. 1997. *The Stark Reality of Stretching*. Richmond, BC: Stark Reality Publishing.

Swami Buddhananda. 1998. *Moola Bandha*.
Varanasi, UP, India: Bhargava Bhushan Press.

Swami Sivananada. 1979. *Fourteen Lessons on Raja Yoga*. Himalayas,
India: The Divine Life Society.

Thomson, Arthur. 1964. *A Handbook of Anatomy for Art Students*. 5th edition.
Toronto: General Publishing Company.

Todd, M. 1993. *The Thinking Body*.
Brooklyn, NY: Dance Horizons.

continue your education

ONLINE EDUCATION
Anatomy and Asana: Monthly Ezine to Your Email Account

This is a free ezine to help continue to develop your understanding of anatomy and asana. Each month we look at a topic of anatomy and apply it to asana – a good burst of knowledge to incorporate into your practice and teaching.

To receive our free monthly ezine on a topic of anatomy as it relates to yoga asana, please visit our website at www.anatomyandasana.com (Like you, we don't like SPAM. We do not sell, trade, or in any way share your email address. It is used to send you your anatomy and asana and to provide you with updates on upcoming courses and workshops).

LIVE WORKSHOPS
Anatomy and Asana

Hundreds of participants have learned principles of anatomy and asana from Susi Hately Aldous. She ignites audiences with her passion, and her enthusiasm is contagious, making anatomy fun and easy to learn. Susi Hately Aldous serves up a combination of simple to understand, easy to apply information that can be used in your classes immediately. Her experiential workshops range from three-hour sessions to weekend intensives to five weekly sessions.

Anatomy and Asana – The Basics

Understanding the fundamentals of anatomy and physiology will help you be a great teacher. With these fundamentals, you will be able to answer many of the questions your students ask, offer them suggestions to enhance their practice, and be able to switch up your cueing to ensure all of your students understand and feel the asana they are practicing.

You will learn:

- How to use anatomical language to enhance your understanding of body movement
- A step-by-step process for understanding the connections between the head, neck, and shoulders and how they anatomically bring lightness and grace in inversions, back bends, forward bends, twists, and standing poses
- A step-by-step process for understanding the connections between the lower back, hips, knees, and feet and how they anatomically work together to create ease, strength, and stability in standing poses, back bends, forward bends, twists, and inversions
- How to excite or calm the nervous system with different yoga techniques
- How to use breath and bandhas to bring strength, stability, and ease to all of the yoga asanas
- What fascia is and how it impacts movement into and out of asanas
- A proven way to explain anatomical concepts so that you inspire and engage your students to go deeper into their practice

Anatomy and Asana – Preventing Yoga Injuries

Yoga offers an incredible way to improve and maintain your health and well-being. Since hatha yoga is exercise, injuries are possible. This workshop will give you strategies and principles that you can use to help your students prevent yoga-related injuries, and if they have already occurred, what you can do to help your students overcome them.

Here is a portion of what you will learn:

- The eight steps for an injury-free yoga practice
- The hidden anatomical reason for almost all injuries in yoga
- How to prevent knee and hip injuries
- Why hamstring strains occur
- How to create mobility and stability of the spine to reduce back and neck injuries
- How to offset carpal tunnel syndrome and repetitive strain injuries to the elbows and wrists
- Five steps to help a student recover from a yoga-related injury

To book or for further details…

call: **403.229.2617**
email: **iloveanatomy@anatomyandasana.com**

Or visit our website at **www.anatomyandasana.com**

TESTIMONIAL

Stephanie Adams, *RYT, Senior Trainer, Author and Creator "YogaFit Kids"*

"After 10 years of study and teaching, including numerous conferences, workshops and teacher trainings, this is the most innovative workshop relating to asana that I have taken. I received a truly deeper understanding of how human biomechanics work in these poses, and, more importantly, how often we might not be doing these poses in a way that serves our bodies best. Susi teaches us real, practical and experiential methods for reteaching the body to move in the way it was designed to. Susi's truly inovative and accepting approach and easy-to-understand teaching style is truly enlightening. I highly recommend this workshop for every yoga instructor, master, or teacher trainer no matter what your style or approach."

Anatomy and Asana is absolutely lovely. Both informative and very calming.

— *Lorrie Maffey, **Physiotherapist***

This book is very easy to follow. It has a superb foundation and depth of knowledge along with practical applications.

— *Jennifer Steed, **Founder: Trinity Yoga Teacher Training Program***

I found this to be a lovely book that is easy to read, interesting, entertaining and educating. If every yoga instructor and enthusiast was to read and utilize this book, students would be able to experience connections that they never thought possible.

— *Suzette O'Byrne, **Yoga Instructor***

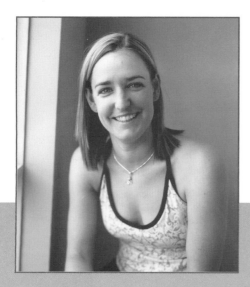

About the Author

Susi Hately Aldous is the facilitator of the Anatomy and Asana workshop series taught around Canada and the United States. She is also the author of the globally read Anatomy and Asana ezine, a monthly e-lesson that explains concepts of anatomy as they relate to yoga asanas. Her diverse background, which includes a BSc. Kinesiology, Yoga Certification and practical experience in physical rehabilitation, provides a functional and common sense approach to her teaching. Her students say that her style is engaging, empowering, and loads of fun.

Susi lives in Calgary, Alberta, where she owns and operates Functional Synergy, a yoga therapy studio that specializes in designing custom yoga programs for people with injury or illness.

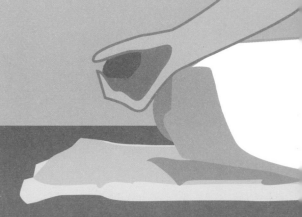

Anatomy and Asana:
Preventing Yoga Injuries

ISBN-13: 978-0-939616-54-1
ISBN-10: 0-939616-54-8

Published by **Eastland Press (Seattle)**
www.eastlandpress.com

9 780939 616541 >

Printed in China